ETHICS
AND
BASIC LAW
For Medical Imaging Professionals

ETHICS AND BASIC LAW
For Medical Imaging Professionals

Bettye G. Wilson, MEd, RT(R)(CT), RDMS
Associate Professor, Radiologic Sciences
Division of Medical Imaging and Therapy
Department of Diagnostic and Critical Care
School of Health Related Professions
The University of Alabama at Birmingham
Birmingham, Alabama

 F. A. DAVIS COMPANY • Philadelphia

F. A. Davis Company
1915 Arch Street
Philadelphia, PA 19103

Printed in the United States of America

Last digit indicates print number: 10 9 8 7 6 5 4 3 2 1

Publisher: Jean-Francois Vilain
Senior Acquisitions Editor: Lynn Borders Caldwell
Developmental Editor: Crystal Spraggins
Production Editor: Jessica Howie Martin
Cover Designer: Louis J. Forgione

As new scientific information becomes available through basic and clinical research, recommended treatments and drug therapies undergo changes. The author and publisher have done everything possible to make this book accurate, up to date, and in accord with accepted standards at the time of publication. The author, editors, and publisher are not responsible for errors or omissions or for consequences from application of the book, and make no warranty, expressed or implied, in regard to the contents of the book. Any practice described in this book should be applied by the reader in accordance with professional standards of care used in regard to the unique circumstances that may apply in each situation. The reader is advised always to check product information (package inserts) for changes and new information regarding dose and contraindications before administering any drug. Caution is especially urged when using new or infrequently ordered drugs.

Library of Congress Cataloging-in-Publication Data

Ethics and basic law for medical imaging professionals / [edited by]
    Bettye G. Wilson.
        p.   cm.
    Includes bibliographical references and index.
    ISBN 0-8036-0152-2 (pbk.)
    1. Radiography, Medical—Moral and ethical aspects.
    2. Radiography, Medical—Law and legislation—United States.
    I. Wilson, Bettye G.
        [DNLM: 1. Radiology—standards—United States. 2. Ethics,
    Professional—United States. 3. Diagnostic Imaging—United States-
    -legislation.   WN 21 E84 1997]
    RC78.E84   1997
    174'.2—dc21
    DNLM/DLC
    for Library of Congress   96-53384

This book is dedicated with unending love and appreciation to my parents, the late George Evans and Velma Simmons Greene.

Preface

Textbooks on ethics in health care, although numerous, tend to address the topic as it relates to either medicine (doctors and nurses) or other specific disciplines. No text specifically addresses medical imaging, to any large degree. Law texts, until recently, were guilty of the same omissions.

Ethics and Basic Law for Medical Imaging Professionals was written to assist educators, professional practitioners, and students of medical imaging in learning ethics and basic law applicable to the profession. My idea for the text began as I was pursuing a baccalaureate degree and stayed with me as I pursued my master's degree. Further fodder for the development of this text was provided by D. Gay Golded Utz, MEd, ARRT(R) and Mary E. Guy, PhD, two instructors of ethics at the University of Alabama at Birmingham, where I studied. (Dr. Guy is the author of *Ethical Decision Making in Everyday Work Situations* published by Quorum Books.)

This text is my answer to the problems I have encountered throughout my career. The book contains discipline-specific material to foster the reader's grasp of the history of ethics and how personal ethics can be developed. Professional codes of conduct or ethics are presented and then dissected so that they are better understood. Step-by-step ethical problem-solving techniques should guide the reader in solving both simple and complex ethical problems.

Discussion questions, included in each chapter of the text, are designed to encourage thought and interaction. The text contains both actual legal cases and case studies written by the contributors based on their professional experience. These cases not only encourage but implore the readers to apply the principles discussed in the text, thereby provoking critical thinking and debate. Unique features of this text include chapters on charting and documentation, chemically dependent colleagues, and administrative ethics. The chapter on informed consent should be of special interest to medical imaging professionals, especially during this time of changes in job roles (job descriptions). Educators may find the section on consent for human experimentation useful, since most of us are now requested to do more and more research, especially those of us in university settings.

The chapters on law are provided to specifically address legal issues, some of which may also contain ethical elements pertinent to medical imaging.

It is my desire that the aforementioned highlights will make a significant positive impact on the level of ethics knowledge in people who are professionally linked with medical imaging.

Bettye G. Wilson

Acknowledgments

This book would not have been possible without the support and encouragement of many people. Very special thanks to Maria Carter Tyson, a very talented and special person. Maria performed all of the word processing tasks for the text. She deciphered my scribble and laughed at my mistakes while lifting my spirits and encouraging me every step of the way. Dr. Charles Joiner, Dean of the School of Health Related Professions at the University of Alabama at Birmingham, is always a source of support and encouragement to me. The faculty and staff within the Division of Medical Imaging and Therapy all encourage each other in good times and bad. Associate Professor Paula Pate-Schloeder, College Misericordia, Dallas, Pennsylvania, is a kindred spirit and shared her knowledge willingly. The staff at F. A. Davis, especially Lynn Borders Caldwell and Crystal Spraggins, were pure joy to work with. Their professional qualities are outstanding. I truly believe this experience was enjoyable because of them.

Finally, I must give thanks to my siblings, Marie, Helen, and Fred; and my siblings-in-law, Mary, Audretta, and Ross, for their support and continued practice of and adherence to the fine ethical standards and values instilled in us by our parents, to whom this text is dedicated. My husband Willie deserves a huge thanks for his encouragement and patience. My daughter Kassaundra and son Byronn have never wavered in their love for me. The love and faith of all three keeps me going. Byronn, a senior Art Studio major with emphasis in Graphic Design, was my consultant for the design and content of charts and figures for this text and other projects. Kassaundra, a senior Social Psychology major, practices her psychology skills on me to get me going when I'm in a slump.

To all those mentioned and to those I may have inadvertently forgotten, many, many thanks.

BGW

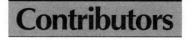
Contributors

Sharon B. Barnes, MPH, ARRT(R)
Clinical Coordinator and Instructor
Radiologic Technology Program
Jefferson State Community College
Birmingham, Alabama

Norman E. Bolus, BS, CNMT
Teacher, Nuclear Medicine
  Technology Program
School of Health Related Professions
University of Alabama at
  Birmingham
Birmingham, Alabama

Steven B. Dowd, EdD, ARRT(R)
Program Director and Associate
  Professor
Director, Radiography Program
Division of Medical Imaging and
  Therapy
School of Health Related Professions
University of Alabama at
  Birmingham
Birmingham, Alabama

Michael W. Drafke, MS, ARRT(R)
Professor of Business, Marketing,
  and Management
Formerly Program Director
Department of Radiology
College of DuPage
Glen Ellyn, Illinois

**Jane Faulkner Evans, JD,
  ARRT(R)(NMT)**
Evans and Wallace, Attorneys at Law
Birmingham, Alabama

Rebecca W. Lam, MEd, ARRT(R)
Associate Professor
Department of Radiologic
  Technologies
School of Allied Health Sciences
Medical College of Georgia
Augusta, Georgia

**Bettye G. Wilson, MEd, RT(R)(CT),
  RDMS**
Associate Professor, Radiologic
  Sciences
Division of Medical Imaging and
  Therapy
Department of Diagnostic and
  Critical Care
School of Health Related Professions
The University of Alabama at
  Birmingham
Birmingham, Alabama

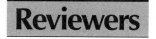

Reviewers

Joseph Bittengle, MEd, BS, RT(R)
Chairman and Assistant Professor
Department of Radiologic
  Technology
University of Arkansas for Medical
  Sciences
Little Rock, Arkansas

Kathryn S. Durand, RT(R), AS
Program Director
Radiologic Technology Program
School of Radiologic Technology
Lawrence and Memorial Hospital
New London, Connecticut

Michael Lee Fugate, MEd, RT(R)
Lead Didactic Faculty
Radiography Program
Santa Fe Community College
Gainesville, Florida

Arthur W. Kroetz, MA, RT(R)
Department Chair
School of Allied Health Professions
Department of Radiologic
  Technology
Loma Linda University
Loma Linda, California

**Millicent B. Nicholas, MSW, BS,
  RT(R)**
Assistant Professor
Radiography Education
Middlesex County College
Edison, New Jersey

Elizabeth Price, RT(R)(M)(CT), BS
Program Director
School of Radiologic Technology
Community General Hospital
Reading, Pennsylvania

Milton Schwartzberg, JD
Private Practice
Boston, Massachusetts

Kathleen E. Valetsky, EDM
Director
Radiography Program
York Health System
York, Pennsylvania

Contents

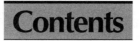

FIVE

Patient Consent   51
Steven B. Dowd, EdD, ARRT(R)

SIX

The Chemically Dependent Colleague   72
Rebecca W. Lam, MEd, ARRT(R)

TEN

Medical Legal Issues for the Practice of Medical Imaging   **151**

Sharon B. Barnes, MPH, ARRT(R)
Steven B. Dowd, EdD, ARRT(R)
Jane Faulkner Evans, JD, ARRT(R)(NMT)

ELEVEN
Administrative Ethics

164

Steven B. Dowd, EdD, ARRT(R)
Michael W. Drafke, MS, ARRT(R)

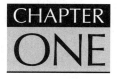

An Introduction to Ethics

Bettye G. Wilson, MEd, RT(R)(CT), RDMS

The news media are constantly bombarding the public with information regarding the ethics of public officials and people in the health professions. However, some confusion exists as to what ethics really means and where it had its origin.

The purpose of this chapter is to provide the reader with information regarding the history of ethics and the persons who are credited with the most-cited theories of ethical behavior. It also provides a modern perspective on ethics.

OBJECTIVES

At the end of this chapter, the reader will be able to:
- Describe the evolution of medical ethics from a historical standpoint
- Name the individuals credited with formulating traditional ethical theories
- Define the traditional ethical theories
- Provide an example of a modern perspective on ethical theory

HISTORICAL PERSPECTIVE

Ethics may well have begun in prehistoric times. Consciously or unconsciously, prehistoric humans began to consider their own ethical behavior and that of others when cooperative interactions occurred. The individual behaviors of members of a group affected the well-being of the group as a whole. This necessitated the regulation of ethical behaviors of the group members. Primitive standards of ethical behavior developed after taboos were violated, out of habitual behavior that became custom, or from laws set forth by the leader or leaders of a group.[1]

Pythagoras, a sixth-century Greek philosopher, is credited with developing one of the earliest known moral philosophies. He postulated that, to have a good life, one should be devoted to mental discipline. He also advocated simplicity in dress, food, and speech. Pythagoras initiated the idea of "divinely inspired personal mortality" and is said to have influenced the development of the Hippocratic Oath,[2] which could be considered one of the first professional codes of ethics.

Credited to Hippocrates, a Greek physician who lived from around 460 to 375 B.C., the Hippocratic Oath was first written in the fifth century B.C. Sometime during the tenth or eleventh century, the oath became Christianized to eliminate references to pagan gods.[3] The oath focuses on the physician's duty to the patient and to the other members of the health care profession.[4]

The Code of Hammurabi was an even earlier attempt to regulate medicine for the protection of the patient. It was formulated in Babylonia in 1727 B.C. Around this same time, the Egyptians also sought to regulate the practice of medicine for the good of the patient. *The Book of Toth* admonishes Egyptian physicians to abide by the prescription for medical practice or face the penalty of death.[5] The first attempt at establishing both cognitive and character attributes desirable in a good physician can be identified in ancient Persian medical ethics.[6] The Persian medical ethics and the Hippocratic corpus provided the thread from which the fabric of modern medical codes of ethics and conduct was woven.

The writings of ancient Greek philosophers, especially Plato, are seen as precursors of later theories on ethics. In *The Republic*, Plato presented his theory on morality. He surmised that if people act morally, they are happy, and people generally desire happiness. In their quest for this happiness, they will strive to do what is considered morally correct. Plato's theory can be debated on the grounds that not all persons desire happiness to the same degree, or even know what true happiness is. However, while debatable, Plato's theory on morality provided a basis for thought on the influence morality has on human behavior.

In the 13th century, Saint Thomas Aquinas provided the world with an ethical theory based on religion. The Natural Law Theory of the Roman Catholic Church, as put forth by Aquinas, stated that people could discover moral principles, which may be described as objective truths, simply by exploring the nature of things and applying reason. According to Aquinas, the ability to reason is a unique God-given trait. Among all living creatures, only humans have this ability. Therefore, according to Aquinas, God has instilled morality within human beings as part of human nature. This morality should guide humans in their quest to preserve life, propagate the species, and search for truth and a peaceful society. Moral law, as defined by Aquinas, is based on human beings' inherent inclinations and ability to use the power of reason when deciding the correct course of conduct. Saint Thomas Aquinas's natural law ethics is reported to be the basis for most biomedical issues.[7]

During the 14th century, numerous plagues struck the European continent.[8] The aftermath of those plagues found physicians examining their moral duties toward their patients. Guilds were formed that influenced the development of physician education and qualifications, peer-review boards, licensure and board certification, and other aspects still in existence today.[2]

The 16th century saw accelerated growth in the exploration of ethics by numerous theorists and the development of traditional ethical theories. Francis Bacon (1561–1626) divided the practice of medicine into three distinct areas: (1) the preservation of health, (2) the cure of disease, and (3) the prolongation of life. Shortly after Bacon's revelation of his divisions of medicine, physicians declared the prolongation of life to be the prime function of medicine. As an extension of Bacon's work, Rodericus Castro (1546–1627) authored *The Responsible Physician or The Duties of the Physician Towards the Public*. This text is considered one of the premiere works on medical ethics.[2]

Sir Isaac Newton (1643–1727), an English mathematician and philosopher; David Hume (1711–1776), a Scottish philosopher and historian; Immanuel Kant (1724–1804), a German philosopher; and John Stuart Mill (1806–1873), an English philosopher and political economist are credited with advances in the study of ethics from the 17th through the 19th centuries.[2] Newton applied scientific principles to problem solving, leading to a scientific rather than a moral focus in medicine. Hume, considered a communitarian, contributed to redirecting ethical theory toward the creation of community associations, the promotion of public health, and the development of national goals for the benefit of the masses.[9] Immanuel Kant, Jeremy Bentham, and Bentham's student John Stuart Mill are credited with developing two of the most common traditional ethical theories, deontology and utilitarianism (see section on ethical theories below).

The study of ethics and the formulation of ethical theory have continued into the 20th century. Particularly noteworthy contributions have been made by two professors of philosophy, W. D. Ross of Oxford University and John Rawls of Harvard. Ross developed a set of rules geared specifically toward governing professional behaviors. These rules are based on the fulfillment of professional duties. Rawls, on the other hand, used the strengths and weaknesses of common ethical theories to derive a set of principles providing equal liberty for all while addressing the needs of the less fortunate.[10] Both of these men have seen their philosophies referenced by others, especially those formulating ethical policies and codes in medicine.

ETHICAL THEORIES

Webster's New World Dictionary[11] defines "theory" as an idea formulated following verifiable observation of some phenomenon. Ethical theories are formulated in that same manner and are introduced as a means of helping in the understanding of moral behavior. The traditional ethical theories are generally divided into two schools of thought, deontology and teleology (Fig. 1–1).

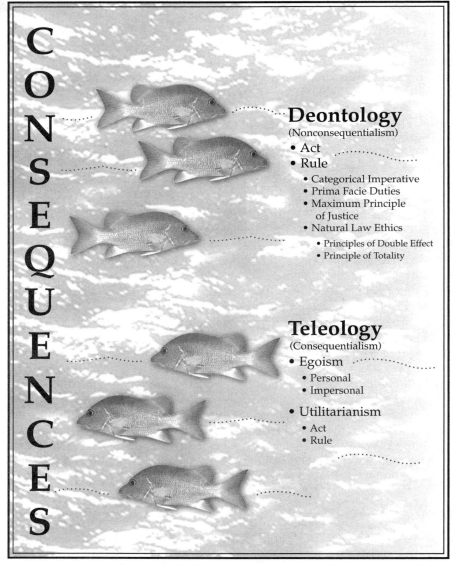

FIGURE 1–1. Deontology and teleology.

Deontology

Deontology, in its purest form, was developed by Immanuel Kant. In his theory, Kant sought to exclude the consideration of consequences when making moral decisions or performing moral acts. According to Kant, nothing is good in and of itself except a "good will." He defined "will" as the unique human ability to act according to principles (laws). The concept of duty is also contained within Kant's theory of good will. Kant based his theory on Saint Thomas Aquinas's natural law ethics, which defined humans as rational beings, with their morality based on the uniquely human capacity to reason.

Deontologists believe that morality is based on reason, and that principles derived from reason are universal and should be held as universal truths. Kant, in an effort to supply these universal truths, assembled what is known as Kant's Categorical Imperative, which states that "we should act in such a way as to will the maxim of our action to become universal law."[12] *Webster's New World Dictionary*[11] defines "maxim" as a concisely expressed principle or rule of conduct, or a statement of a general truth.

The maxim attributed to Kant that has relevance to health care is this: "We must always treat others as ends and not as means only." Healthcare professionals adhering to this position would never view their role of providing care to a patient as just a job for which one receives pay, but would view each patient as a person to whom a professional duty is owed. Since deontology is a duty-based ethical theory, it may also be referred to as nonconsequentialism. There are two categories of nonconsequential/deontological ethical theories: act and rule.

Act Nonconsequentialism

Act nonconsequentialism mandates that each act or action should be evaluated individually to ascertain whether it is right or wrong. This theory holds that there are no rules or guidelines to govern our behavior; the situation governs the act or action. Each situation must be seen and evaluated as a unique ethical dilemma.

Rule Nonconsequentialism

Rule nonconsequentialism maintains that there are one or more rules, which may be derived from the nature of a situation, which serve as the moral standards for ethical decision making. While others may exist, there are generally four accepted positions on rule nonconsequentialism: the categorical imperative (discussed earlier in this chapter), prima facie duties, the maximin principle of justice, and natural law ethics.

Prima Facie Duties. Prima facie duties are attributed to W. D. Ross. In an attempt to unite specific aspects of nonconsequentialism with those of utilitarianism (see section on teleological ethical theories), Ross determined that, in deciding between ethical alternatives to a problem, the options must be weighed according to the duties that would be fulfilled by performing or not performing each option. Then a decision must be made regarding which of the duties the individual is most obliged to perform.[7] As a guide to solving ethical problems, Ross cited six categories of prima facie duties. These are:

1. Duties of fidelity
2. Duties of gratitude
3. Duties of justice
4. Duties of beneficence
5. Duties of self-improvement
6. Duties of maleficence

Ross described prima facie duties as being intuitive and conditional.[13] He defined intuition as being simply the feeling within that an act or action is right. Prima facie duties are conditional in that they can be overridden and still retain their character as duties.[7] What is interesting about Ross's list of prima facie duties is that these same duties are referred to as principles of biomedical ethics by numerous authors. Whether alluded to as "principles" or "duties," they are intended to create what has been described as a framework on which a solid structure of ethical decisions can be built.[14] These duties or principles also provide the foundation for the codes of ethics and/or conduct that govern the ethical behavior of health-care professionals.

Maximin Principle of Justice. The maximin principle of justice was formulated by John Rawls, a Harvard professor of philosophy, in an effort to find a workable solution to problems of social morality.[7] Termed the "maximin principle" because it attempts to maximize the lot of those who are minimally advantaged, its focus is on the establishment of principles of justice.[15]

Rawls envisioned a hypothetical state of nature called the "original position." In this position, individuals are not aware of their talents or socioeconomic condition; all are similar in capacities, interests, and needs. Rawls theorized that if people in the original position were asked to formulate a principle that would guarantee justice for all, they would choose two: difference and liberty.

The difference principle does not allow inequality unless it is advantageous to everyone and arises under conditions of equal opportunity. The liberty principle asserts that all those participating in or affected by an act or action should have equal opportunity to the greatest amount of liberty possible. These two principles form Rawls's maximin principle of justice and are applicable to health care in the allocation of scarce resources.

Natural Law Ethics. The Roman Catholic interpretation is said to be the moral standpoint from which to view biomedical issues. Attributed to Saint Thomas Aquinas, natural law ethics is an interpretation of natural law theory, which is a general opinion that "moral principles are objective truths which can be discovered in the nature of things by reason alone."[16] Saint Thomas

Aquinas's view on natural law contains rules of conduct based on God-given inclinations inherent within the nature of every human. According to Aquinas, God's intentions for humans are preservation of life, propagation of the species, education of the progeny, and pursuit of truth and a peaceful society. Humankind is able to carry out these intentions because God has endowed the human species with the ability to reason. Thus, when we act according to reason, we act in accordance with the nature of humankind; if we act contrary to reason, it is both unnatural and immoral.[17]

DISCUSSION QUESTION
List several current ethical issues in medicine. Citing his theory on natural law ethics, what do you think Saint Thomas Aquinas's view would be on each issue?

The theory of natural law ethics as developed by Aquinas is based on several principles. Those having particular applications in medicine are the principle of double effect and the principle of totality.[18]

PRINCIPLE OF DOUBLE EFFECT. The principle of double effect is intended to help make choices easier when we are faced with an act or action that will produce both bad and good effects. Simply, the principle of double effect tells us that an act or action should be performed only if the intention is to bring about the good effect and only if the bad effect is unintended or an indirect consequence. For an action to meet the criteria of the principle of double effect, the following four conditions must be satisfied:

1. The act or action itself must be morally neutral or good.
2. The good effect must be the only intention.
3. The good effect must be equal to or greater in importance than the bad effect.
4. The bad effect must not be the means by which the good effect is accomplished.[7]

DISCUSSION QUESTION
You suspect that one of your pediatric patients is the victim of non-accidental trauma (child abuse). If you report your suspicions to the proper authorities, your state laws mandate that the child be removed from the care of the parents until an investigation of the allegations is complete. What good effect is hoped for in this situation? What bad effect may be a consequence of reporting your suspicions? Does your reporting of the action satisfy the four conditions necessary for application of the principle of double effect?

PRINCIPLE OF TOTALITY. The principle of totality asserts that human beings have the right to dispose of their organs or destroy their capacity to function *only* if the general overall health of the body demands it.

DISCUSSION QUESTION
Apply the principle of totality to procedures such as hysterectomy, tubal ligation, and vasectomy for contraceptive purposes. Under this principle, are these procedures unethical?

Teleology

Teleological ethical theories deem that the consequences of an act or action should be the main focus when deciding what course of action should be undertaken to solve an ethical problem. In following teleological leanings, the best solution would be the one producing the greatest amount of happiness or the least amount of unhappiness.[19] In essence, teleological ethical theory holds that the ends justify the means.[20] Because teleology focuses on the consequences of an act or action, these theories may also be referred to as consequential ethical theories. The two most notable types of consequential ethical theories are egoism and utilitarianism.

Egoism

The aim of egoism is the promotion of the best long-term interests of the individual. For an act or action to be considered moral, it must produce a greater ratio of good to evil for the individual, over an extended period of time, than any of the available alternatives. Egoism may be divided further into two types: personal and impersonal.

Personal. Personal egoists pursue their own best long-term interests. They wish to protect themselves from bad consequences, so they carefully choose the act or action that produces the greatest amount of good to benefit them personally. They believe in self-protection but make no attempt at proposing what other individuals should do.

Impersonal. Impersonal egoists believe that everyone should choose the act or action that promotes his or her best interests over the long term.

Because health-care professionals exist to serve others, egoism in either form is viewed as incompatible.[7]

Utilitarianism

Attributed to the work of philosophers Jeremy Bentham and his student John Mill, utilitarianism simply holds that we should act to produce the greatest ratio of good to evil for all concerned. Utilitarianism has been identified as the consequential or teleological ethical theory applicable to moral decisions in health care. According to Bentham's philosophy, actions are right to the extent that they promote happiness and pleasure for everyone concerned, and wrong to the degree that they produce pain and no pleasure. The "pleasure" described by Bentham is synonymous with good. Like most ethical theories, utilitarianism may be divided into two categories: act and rule.

Act Utilitarianism. Act utilitarianism asserts that the correct act is the one that produces the greatest ratio of good to bad. An act utilitarian, when contemplating a solution to an ethical problem, will generally ask, "What good and bad consequences will result from this action in this circumstance?"[9] No specific moral rules are considered by the act utilitarian, only the act or action itself.

Rule Utilitarianism. Rule utilitarianism decrees that we should base our actions on the consequences of the rule or rules under which an act or action falls, not on the consequences of the act or action itself. The rules in rule utilitarianism may be those offered by religious beliefs, such as the Ten Commandments; those offered by professional codes of ethics or conduct; those set forth by professional groups in the best interest of their clients, like the American Hospital Association's *A Patient's Bill of Rights;* or an arbitrary set of beliefs held by an individual.

DISCUSSION QUESTION
Think of what you perceive as an ethical problem you have encountered, or may encounter, within your scope of practice as a medical imaging professional. What act or action did you choose, or would you choose, in solving the problem? Now apply both act and rule utilitarianism to your solution. On which theory was your solution based? How do you know?

A MODERN PERSPECTIVE ON ETHICS: BIOETHICS

As anyone exposed to mass communication knows, ethics is a hot topic. People holding or aspiring to political office are subject to ethical scrutiny, as are those who hold lesser positions in public employment. The majority of states have enacted laws or statutes seeking to govern the ethical conduct of public employees and elected or appointed political figures.

Associations governing college sports have issued sanctions against institutions found in violation of ethical guidelines governing the players and administration. Just about every profession has guidelines for professional ethical behavior of those in practice; medicine is no exception.

Bioethics, developed in the early 1960s, is specifically devoted to addressing ethical problems in medical practice, the delivery of health care, and medical and biological research.[21] Bioethics is often viewed as a response to the rapid growth and technological advancements in health care. Issues such as abortion, euthanasia, HIV and drug testing, in vivo and in vitro fertilization, organ retrieval and implantation, genetic testing and engineering, surrogate parenthood, and allocation of scarce resources often present unique ethical and legal problems in health care.

The American Hospital Association[22] defines bioethics, or biomedical ethics, as "the study of rational processes for determining the most morally desirable course of action in the face of conflicting value choices associated with the practice of medicine." Bioethics seeks to resolve conflicts in medicine when there are desires from several sources and all cannot be met. Researchers, physicians, and patients may differ significantly in their religious or moral beliefs. The challenge of bioethics is to achieve and maintain a delicate balance between the rights of the individual and the needs of society.[23]

Health-care distribution in the United States occurs at both the microallocation and macroallocation levels. Because of this, two newer forms of bioethics have surfaced: microethics and macroethics.

Microethics

Microallocation involves the determination of who will receive scarce resources such as intensive care beds and dialysis services, and it involves solving problems dealing with matters such as abortion, feeding tubes, and ventilators. The determination for the use of a specific resource and who will receive that resource is made by the physician and is said to be a microethical determination. It is based on the interpersonal ethical relationship of the patient and the physician.

Macroethics

In contrast, macroallocation occurs at a much higher level. Generally, decisions on macroallocation are made by Congress, state legislatures, insurance companies, private foundations, and health-care organizations.[24] Macroallocation determinations are made for all individuals within a certain group regardless of the types of individuals making up the group.[2] Norman Daniels[25] has identified several questions that must be answered by those making determinations on the macroallocation level. They are:

1. What kinds of health-care services will exist in a society?
2. Who will receive them and on what basis?

3. Who will deliver them?
4. How will the burdens of financing them be distributed?
5. How will the power and control of these services be distributed?

Ethical decisions made at the macroallocation level are macroethical decisions, and as such require the application of justice. A general definition of justice is the treatment of all with fairness and equality. Or, according to Aristotle, justice consists of giving each human his or her due.[26] John Rawls put forth his notion of justice as follows:

1. Justice guarantees maximum freedom to every member of the community.
2. Justice guarantees persons with similar skills and abilities equal access to offices and positions.
3. Justice guarantees a distribution (of goods and services) for the maximum benefit of the poorest persons.[15]

Macroethical concerns are justified in this era of change associated with the rising cost of health care and the advancements in health-care technology.

DISCUSSION QUESTION
Which type of ethical concern (microethical or macroethical) is each of the following and why?

1. Medicare
2. Organ transplantation
3. HIV testing program
4. Abortion

The Centers for Disease Control and Prevention, the National Institutes of Health, the Office of Technology Assessment, and the United States Supreme Court are but a few of the agencies involved in the development and issuance of laws, policies, rules, and decisions concerning health care at the macro level. These agencies regularly use ethical premises and standards in their work.[7]

To further help resolve ethical problems on the macro and micro levels, medical ethicists founded the Hastings Center in Hastings-on-Hudson in 1969 and the Kennedy Institute of Ethics at Georgetown University in Washington, D.C., in 1971.[23] Major university medical centers have hired medical ethicists and formed hospital ethics committees to assist physicians, other health-care professionals, staff, and patients with health-care decisions involving ethical considerations. Never in the history of health care have so many people been aware of the ethical problems associated with such care and committed to finding workable ethical solutions to these problems.

Health-care professionals use their personal value system and professional ethics, as prescribed by their professional codes of ethics or conduct, in solving ethical problems. Another term for professional ethics is "applied ethics," the purpose of which is to guarantee professional ethical conduct in the pursuit of health, the prevention of death, and the alleviation of suffering.[24] Several principles have been developed to assist the health-care professional in the determination of right and wrong. These principles are invaluable to the health-care professional involved in ethical decision making and will be presented in Chapter 4.

CONCLUSION

Ethics and ethical concerns continue to grow in importance to those of us in health care. Of value in the understanding of ethics is its history, the evolution of ethical theory, and the theorists who formulated what may be viewed as the foundation of current thought. Medical ethics will continue to be a major focus of health care as technical advancements in diagnosis and treatment are made. Medical imaging professionals will not be spared the rigors of ethical decision making or the demands of performing their jobs in an ethical manner. A thorough understanding of ethics will enable practitioners to meet this challenge.

REFERENCES

1. Phillips, RS, (ed): Funk & Wagnalls New Encyclopedia, Volume 9. New York, Funk & Wagnalls, Inc., 1985.
2. Loewy, EH: Textbook of Medical Ethics. New York, Plenum, 1989.
3. Lewis, MA, and Tamparo, CD: Medical Law, Ethics, and Bioethics in the Medical Office, ed 3. Philadelphia, FA Davis, 1993.
4. Carroll, C: Legal Issues and Ethical Dilemmas in Respiratory Care. Philadelphia, FA Davis, 1996.
5. Garrison, FH: An Introduction to the History of Medicine. Philadelphia, WB Saunders, 1929.
6. Carrick, P: Medical Ethics in Antiquity. Boston, Reidel, 1985.
7. Barry, VE: Moral Aspects of Health Care. Belmont, CA, Wadsworth, 1982.
8. Amundsen, DW: Medical deontology and the pestilential disease in the later Middle Ages. J Historical Medicine 32:403–421, 1977.
9. Beauchamp, TL, and Childers, JF: Principles of Biomedical Ethics, ed 4. New York, Oxford University Press, 1994.
10. Monagle, JF, and Thomasma, DC: Medical Ethics: A Guide for Health Professionals. Rockville, MD, Aspen, 1988.
11. Webster's New World Dictionary, ed 2. New York, Simon & Schuster, 1982.
12. Kant, I: Groundwork of the Metaphysics of Morals. Translated by JJ Patton. New York, Harper and Row, 1964.
13. Ross, WD: The Right and the Good. Oxford, England, Oxford University Press, 1930.
14. Adler, AM, and Carlton, RR: Introduction of Radiography and Patient Care. Philadelphia, WB Saunders, 1994.
15. Rawls, J: A Theory of Justice. Cambridge, MA, Harvard University Press, 1971.
16. Hughes, CJ: Natural Law. Journal of Medical Ethics 2(1):34–36, 1976.
17. Barcalow, E: Moral Philosophy Theory and Issues. Belmont, CA, Wadsworth, 1994.
18. Munson, R: Intervention and Reflection: Basic Issues in Medical Ethics. Belmont, CA, Wadsworth, 1979.

19. Monagle, JF, and Thomasma, DC: Medical Ethics: A Guide for Health Professionals. Rockville, MD, Aspen, 1988.
20. Purtilo, R: Ethical Dimensions in the Health Professions, ed 2. Philadelphia, WB Saunders, 1993.
21. Bailey, DM, and Schwartzberg, SL: Ethical and Legal Dilemmas in Occupational Therapy. Philadelphia, FA Davis, 1995.
22. American Hospital Association: A Patient's Bill of Rights. Chicago, American Hospital Association, 1992.
23. Finn, J, and Marshall, EL: Medical Ethics. New York, Chelsea House, 1990.
24. Edge, RS, and Groves, JR: The Ethics of Health Care. Albany, Delmar, 1994.
25. Daniels, N: Just Health Care. New York, Cambridge University Press, 1985.
26. Aristotle: Nichomachean Ethics. Indianapolis, Bobbs-Merrill, 1962.

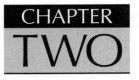

CHAPTER TWO

Developing Personal Ethics

Bettye G. Wilson, MEd, RT(R)(CT), RDMS

Personal ethics plays an important role in the way each of us approaches professional ethical problems and decisions. The purpose of this chapter is to help promote an understanding of the sources from which personal value systems emerge. The assessment of worth is also examined, along with values clarification. Finally, desirable core values and their meanings are discussed and related to ethical issues involving medical imaging professionals.

OBJECTIVES

At the end of this chapter, the reader will be able to:

- Describe the sources of personal values
- List examples of how these sources shape our value system
- Define "values clarification"
- Complete a values clarification exercise to determine which personal values are held
- List the ten core values that are necessary in today's health-care environment
- Give examples of the application of the core values to medical imaging

SOURCES OF VALUES

Ethics are based on values. An individual's ethical behavior and the ethical decisions made by that individual may directly relate to his or her personal values. All people do not have the same values, and therefore differ in their ethical behavior.

Values are core beliefs concerning what is intrinsically desirable.[1] They help assess the worth of things that are intangible. Our values underlie the decisions we make in work situations and in our private lives.

Most values are derived from four main sources that influence our personal and professional attitudes:

1. Science
2. Culture
3. Religion
4. Experience[2]

Theories on why we are and what we are have been scientifically explored for hundreds of years. The knowledge gained from scientific research is taught to us in the educational system and has a positive or negative bearing on how we perceive life in general and the human condition.

The culture in which we are raised further shapes our value system. For example, Japanese culture values age and wisdom and holds its elderly citizens in high esteem. In the western hemisphere, however, elderly people are sometimes regarded as weak and defenseless and without worth. Generally, the Japanese believe that elderly people are a valuable knowledge resource and therefore honor them. In the United States, elderly people are more likely to be seen as forgetful, senile, and unable to make any meaningful contributions to society.

An individual's religious beliefs may influence his or her values. In households where members regularly attend church services, a higher dependence on religion as a source of values may be observed. This is probably directly related to exposure to religious doctrine on a regular basis. Parents in these households usually live by the doctrine they have been taught and promote the practice of that doctrine in their offspring. If no members of a household regularly attend church services, exposure to doctrine related to a specific religious denomination may be almost nonexistent. Therefore, members of these households generally differ in the degree to which religion shapes their value system.

As we grow older, life experiences give additional structure to our personal value system. The experience of living in a household or having a family in which all are taught to always do their best in a given situation, and in fact are rewarded for doing so, teaches family members to value productivity and the pursuit of personal goals. If, however, a household or family allows procrastination and less-than-average or mediocre performance, the value system will probably not be as high as that in a more goal-oriented household.

VALUES CLARIFICATION

How can individuals determine their values? One method that may be useful is values clarification. Formulated by Louis Rath, values clarification is designed to help individuals discover, analyze, and prioritize their personal values and to exhibit these values in everyday personal and professional situations. Values clarification helps individuals describe their values, but it does not attempt to prescribe what they should or should not do in a particular situation. In essence, values clarification helps people determine what they value; that is, those things that have worth.

Values clarification allows individuals to choose freely from available alternatives, after they consider the consequences of each alternative placed before them, and to be proud and happy with the choice made. Individuals should also be able to defend and affirm that choice publicly if necessary. They should make the choice part of their general behavior and repeat the choice in situations of the same type.[3] Those who follow this logical order of promoting their values are choosing, prizing, and acting.[2] Under these headings there are seven subprocesses:

Choosing
1. Make the choice without reservation.
2. Select from all alternatives.
3. Select your choice only after careful consideration.

Prizing
4. Be proud of and happy with your choice.
5. Be willing to defend or affirm the choice publicly.

Acting
6. Make the choice part of your behavior.
7. Repeat the choice in similar situations.

The model values clarification exercise that follows is designed to clarify personal values concerning issues in health care and health-care delivery.[4] An exercise of this type allows participants to make a choice and subsequently examine the feelings that influenced the choice. The value of this exercise is enhanced if it is carried out in a group setting where the moral or values orientation of those present varies. The areas examined may be adapted to any other areas desired simply by changing the questions.

VALUES CLARIFICATION EXERCISE

Instructions

In the space provided, place the letter that best describes your position on the statements listed.

A	B	C	D	E
Totally agree	Somewhat agree	Neutral or undecided	Somewhat disagree	Totally disagree

_E_ 1. Fetuses found to have severe handicaps should be aborted.

_C_ 2. The prolongation of life by extraordinary means is always indicated.

_E_ 3. My role as a medical imaging professional skilled in cardiopulmonary resuscitation (CPR) is to resuscitate a patient, without regard to what may have been decided previously.

_A_ 4. I must follow the orders of the radiologist or sonologist without question.

_A_ 5. Elderly persons should be allowed to die with dignity.

_A_ 6. Advances in medical technology have advanced the quality of life.

_D_ 7. Children should not be allowed to become involved in consent for their treatment.

_A_ 8. The patient should leave decisions concerning his or her life or death to family or significant others.

_B_ 9. Children should be allowed to participate in medical experimentation that is not considered harmful, even if it is not personally beneficial to them.

_E_ 10. Correctional institution inmates should be used in scientific medical experiments because they have wronged society and need to contribute something positive.

_D_ 11. It is easier and safer to sterilize men than women.

_E_ 12. Mentally retarded adults should be sterilized.

_E_ 13. Women should only have women physicians to avoid discrimination and sexual harassment.

_C_ 14. When parents refuse to allow a child to receive medical care, the child should be removed from the parents through the action of the court.

_E_ 15. Fetuses should be used in medical research and experimentation.

_E_ 16. Abortion is the right of a woman and any decision should only involve collaboration with her attending physician.

_E_ 17. If an EEG shows a flat pattern for several consecutive days, life support should be withdrawn.

_A_ 18. There is a shortage of health-care providers in many parts of the United States.

_B_ 19. Radiography, sonography, and nuclear medicine technology are subservient medical professions.

_E_ 20. As a medical imaging professional, I must deny my personal philosophy in support of the philosophy of others.

_A_ 21. All health-care consumers, regardless of race, sex, disease process, etc., should be treated humanistically.

_B_ 22. I should give mouth-to-mouth resuscitation to a homeless derelict if needed.

_A_ 23. A disabled child has value.

_A_ 24. All human life has value.

_A_ 25. I should be consulted on decision making regarding ethical issues in my profession.

_E_ 26. Resource allocation committees should decide who receives scarce resources such as hearts.

_C_ 27. The rights of patients should be more important than the rights of society as a whole.

_A_ 28. People should have the right to inform others of the kind of treatment or nontreatment they desire if they ever become so ill that they cannot communicate their desires to others.

_E_ 29. Because the world is overpopulated, women of childbearing age should be sterilized after two successful pregnancies.

_C_ 30. It is the responsibility of developed nations to give health and financial support to undeveloped countries.

_E_ 31. I should totally support the ethical positions taken by my professional organization(s).

_A_ 32. I should support my personal values over those of others.

_E_ 33. Consideration of the values held by patients is a waste of time.

_E_ 34. The *care* component of health-care delivery is not as important as the *cure* component of health-care delivery.

_D_ 35. The primary role of the health-care practitioner in ethical decision making is implementation of the decision.

_E_ 36. I am uncomfortable performing a medical imaging examination on a terminally ill client.

_E_ 37. Children with disabilities should be institutionalized.

_E_ 38. Behavior modification therapy should be mandatory for people in mental health and correctional institutions to make them conform to society's rules.

_E_ 39. The hospital should remove personal possessions from admitted patients so that they will be safe.

__A__ 40. Health-care consumers should have access to their medical records.

__E__ 41. Withholding information from patients concerning their health makes them feel better.

__E__ 42. Dialysis is always available for those who need it.

__C__ 43. Society should be responsible for the cost of extraordinary medical interventions.

__A__ 44. In my role as a medical imaging professional, confidentiality is very important.

__A__ 45. I value the responsibility of my profession.

__A__ 46. Homosexuality is a sin and should be discouraged.

__E__ 47. Health-care practitioners have the right to withhold information from a patient if that will facilitate medical research using human subjects.

__E__ 48. A patient who refuses treatment once should never receive treatment.

__C__ 49. Organ transplantation should be performed whenever necessary.

$$A = 1, \quad B = 2 \quad C = 3 \quad D = 4 \quad E = 5$$

4|6   3:6   5=15   2:8   22 = 110

Determine the number of 1s, 2s, 3s, 4s, and 5s that you have. Which statements do you seem to have *clear ideas* about?

1. What categories do most of your answers fall under (strongly or somewhat agree, undecided/neutral, or strongly or somewhat disagree)?
2. Is there a pattern to your agreement or disagreement? Are the statements similar? No, similar -
3. Did you uncover an age or sexual bias? No
4. Can you see your value system emerge? Yes.

Some statements in the exercise relate to one another and to certain issues as explained below:

Statement	Issue
5, 8, 16, 17, 28, and 36	Death
11, 12, 16, 29, 46, and 49	Human sexuality and reproduction
3, 4, 19, 20, 25, 31, 35, 44 and 45	Health care and health-care professionals
2, 6, 15, 17, 24, 28, 43, and 50	Advancements in medical technology
1, 7, 9, 14, 23, 37, and 49	Children
9, 10, 15, and 47	Human experimentation

3, 7, 8, 13, 14, 21, 22, 27, 28, 33, 39, 40, 41, 44, and 48	The rights of health-care consumers/clients
9, 10, 27, 29, 30, 32, and 43	The rights of society
18, 26, 40, and 42	Allocation of scarce resources
3, 4, 20, 21, 22, 25, 26, 31, 32, 35, 39, and 45	Obligations

Is there consistency in the way you related to statements dealing with the same issue? NO

What, if any, variables among related statements influenced your decision? NO

What, if anything, did you learn about yourself after completing this exercise? yes

Now, if you have not already done so, discuss the choices of others who performed this exercise.

Be sure that each of them examines and answers all the statements before discussion takes place.

How many of you changed your decision concerning some of the statements after discussion?

How many of you found it easy to stick to your previous decisions after discussion?

Exercise adapted from Steele, SM and Harmon VM: Values Clarification in Nursing. New York, Appleton-Century-Crofts, 1979, pp 70–74, with permission.

The preceding exercise was designed to allow participants to discover some of their personal values. If the group holds many of the same values, then participants probably share very similar cultural backgrounds, religious beliefs, and level of education. Their life experiences may also be parallel. Usually, though, varying values are found in discussion groups simply because it is unusual to find a high number of unrelated individuals, together at one place at a given time with the same values.

CORE VALUES

The difference in values provides the impetus for ongoing disputes over such issues as abortion, euthanasia, and allocation of scarce resources. However, in society, most individuals are expected to possess certain similar values thought to be essential to relations among people.[1,5–8] Ten essential values have been found (Fig. 2–1). Although some of these values may actually overlap, they are "at the core of ethical standards that have survived the ages . . . and when put into practice, these values generate widely recognized virtues that provide benchmarks for ethical decision making."[1]

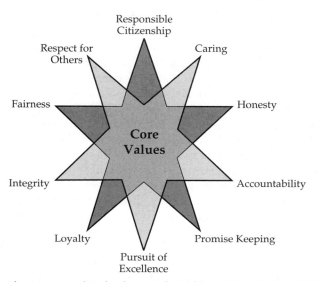

FIGURE 2–1. The ten core ethical values. (Adapted from Mary E. Guy: *Ethical Decision Making in Everyday Work Situations,* reprinted with permission of Quorum Books, an imprint of Greenwood Publishing Group, Inc., Westport, Connecticut. Copyright (c) 1990 by Mary E. Guy. All rights reserved.)

Let's examine the meaning of each core value and relate each one to an ethical issue involving medical imaging professionals.

- **Caring.** Feeling concern or interest for. Probably the most health-care-related of the ten core values, caring is what the delivery of health care is thought to be. A caring medical imaging professional treats every patient with dignity and compassion when called upon to perform a procedure. There is concern for performing one's job to the best of one's ability so that adequate diagnosis may be made and proper treatment provided. It makes no difference to the caring imaging professional whether the patient is young or old, black or white, heterosexual or homosexual; or has a potentially fatal disease process or is in for cataract removal. The caring imaging professional treats all patients as ends in themselves and not simply as means to an end.
- **Honesty.** Refraining from lying, cheating, and stealing; being truthful, trustworthy, sincere, and fair; not deceiving or distorting. The honest medical imaging professional does not lie to the patient. If there is reason to repeat a procedure due to technologist error, the honest imaging professional does not tell the patient that he or she breathed at the wrong time or that the machine didn't work, but explains that, because of technical error, the procedure or projection must be repeated. An honest professional never considers leaving the most

infirm client for others, but proceeds with examinations on a prioritized, or first-come, first-served, basis. No honest professional ever contemplates stealing from a client, but safeguards valuables when required. The honest medical imaging professional endeavors to be sincere and trustworthy so that each client feels secure.

- **Accountability.** Being liable and responsible. Accountable imaging professionals realize that they alone are responsible for conducting the best possible examination or procedure on the patient. They know that if they give 100% to each patient, they have contributed to the diagnosis and treatment process. Accountable imaging professionals are also aware that they may be held liable for injury or adverse reactions resulting from negligent treatment of the patient. They perform examinations within established guidelines so that liability on their part is negligible. For example, an accountable ultrasonographer never leaves the client unattended. He or she is aware that most lawsuits instituted against medical imaging departments are the result of patient falls, usually while the professional is not in attendance.

- **Promise keeping.** Adhering to an agreement, providing a basis for expectations. An imaging professional's acceptance of employment is an agreement, or set of promises, between the employer and employee. The employer promises to pay the employee an agreed amount in exchange for work performed. The employee agrees to perform the services of his or her job description and expects to receive financial remuneration in return. Both must keep their promises in order to maintain a healthy employee-employer relationship. Failure to keep the terms of employment may result in termination by either the employee or employer. Professional codes of conduct or ethics are also binding agreements. The Code of Ethics of the American Society of Radiologic Technologists (ASRT), the Code of Ethics of the Society of Nuclear Medicine Technologists (SNMT), and the Code of Professional Conduct of the Society of Diagnostic Medical Sonographers (SDMS) are the agreements to which radiographers, ultrasonographers, and nuclear medicine technologists are professionally bound. Failure to abide by these codes may result in revocation of the respective registries and loss of professional status. Institutional codes and *A Patient's Bill of Rights* are also binding agreements to which the imaging professional must adhere. These codes will be examined in Chapter Three.

- **Pursuit of excellence.** Following a specified course toward superiority. In medical imaging, this means keeping abreast of current trends in the field and following mandated guidelines specified by the governing body of the profession to which the medical imaging professional belongs. These governing agencies mandate that members of the profession remain proficient in their performance, and toward that end, have specific criteria for continuing education to which members must adhere to maintain active registry status.

- **Loyalty.** Being faithful to ideals. For the medical imaging professional, this value means promoting the values and priorities of the profession. Abiding by the professional code of ethics or conduct governing the behavior of practioners should be foremost in the performance of professional duty. If one cannot, for any reason, remain loyal to one's profession, then an internal examination of why the profession was chosen in the first place is needed. This should aid the practitioner in deciding whether to remain active in the profession or to pursue another to which he or she can remain loyal.
- **Fairness.** Performing duties with justice and honesty; exhibiting open-mindedness and a willingness to admit error; treating all equally. Medical imaging professionals with this value regard all clients (patients) as having equal status. For example, no exceptions are made for those who are known to have more money than others, are more well known, or are relatives of physicians or other health-care providers. In other words, no value is attached to the patient's attributes, but to the patient himself or herself in accordance with established guidelines for treatment and care of all patients.
- **Integrity.** Refraining from self-promotion, avoiding conflicts of interest, and resisting economic pressure. Those possessing this value are faithful to their own beliefs, but do not promote their beliefs over those of their clients. For example, a medical imaging professional has the personal right to a belief that abortion is wrong under any circumstances, but will not refuse to perform a procedure on a client whose opinion on abortion differs or who is about to undergo an abortion.
- **Respect for others.** Showing consideration and concern for others. Recognizing everyone's right to privacy. In health-care delivery, respect for others applies particularly to informed consent. The health-care practitioner who respects others will impart the information necessary for the patient to make informed decisions regarding treatment or nontreatment. The American Hospital Association's *A Patient's Bill of Rights* guarantees the right to informed consent.
- **Responsible citizenship.** Performing one's duties in accordance with societal values. Those stressing this value see it as their duty to report conditions that are against societal values or those of their respective profession. For example, a radiographer has performed numerous procedures on a child in the emergency department on several occasions. The radiographer has noticed that the injuries are consistent with what is now known as nonaccidental trauma (child abuse). The radiographer who values responsible citizenship will report his or her suspicions to the proper authorities, as specified by institutional protocol, without regard for what others think.

From the examination of the ten core values and examples of applications to medical imaging, the importance of these values should be evident. The promotion of the ten values described generates virtues that may aid the practitioner in ethical decision making. You may possess other values that you deem important, and this is acceptable. However, it is desirable that you, as a medical imaging professional, possess at least the ten core values listed. For they, along with the guidelines stressed by your professional code of ethics or conduct, should serve you well by guiding your behavior and forming the foundation from which you may build.

REFERENCES

1. Guy, ME: Ethical Decision Making in Everyday Work Situations. New York, Quorum, 1990.
2. Barry, V: Moral Aspects of Health Care. Belmont, CA, Wadsworth, 1982.
3. Raths, L, Simon, S, and Merrill, H: Values and Teaching. Columbus, OH, Charles E Merrill, 1966.
4. Steele, SM, and Harmon, VM: Values Clarification in Nursing. New York, Appleton-Century-Crofts, 1979.
5. Barry, V: Moral Issues in Business. Belmont, CA, Wadsworth, 1979.
6. Beauchamp, TL, and Bowie, NE: Ethical Theory and Business. Englewood Cliffs, NJ, Prentice-Hall, 1979.
7. Josephson, M: Teaching ethical decision making and principled reasoning. Ethics 1(1):27–33, 1988.
8. Solomon, RC, and Hanson, K: It's Good Business. New York, Atheneum, 1985.

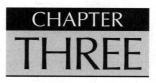

CHAPTER
THREE

Professional Ethics
Examining the
Professional Codes

Norman E. Bolus, BS, CNMT
Steven B. Dowd, EdD, ARRT(R)
Bettye G. Wilson, MEd, RT(R)(CT), RDMS

This chapter reviews the ethical codes set forth by three professional organizations: the Society of Nuclear Medicine–Technologists' Section (SNM–TS), the Society of Diagnostic Medical Sonographers (SDMS), and the American Society of Radiologic Technologists (ASRT). All codes are reprinted with permission from the sources. Each code is analyzed in terms of its meaning to the authors, and the chapter concludes with a brief section on whistle-blowing.

OBJECTIVES

At the end of this chapter, the reader will be able to:
- State the principles contained within each code of ethics
- Give relevant examples of actions corresponding to each code
- Analyze each code
- Describe the relevance of whistle-blowing to the practice of medical imaging

THE USE AND INTENT OF PROFESSIONAL CODES

Ethics focuses on moral questions and guidelines rather than on answers or rules. Thus, Singarella and Salladay[1] have described ethics as a discipline that is *descriptive* rather than *prescriptive* in nature. In previous years, codes were restrictive and told practitioners what they could and could not do. Craig[2] noted that "For many years the health care profession was governed by rigid, no-nonsense rules that discouraged any emotional or personal involvement with patients, and it demanded unquestioning obedience to authority figures." The ASRT Code of Ethics, for example, was extremely restrictive. In 1969, practitioners were forbidden from owning radiographic equipment and could teach their own profession only under the direction of a physician.[3]

Today, most ethical codes focus on the ideals for practice in a profession. These codes establish a foundation for practice instead of telling people what they cannot do. Professional codes of conduct or ethics in health care are written with the basic assumption that practitioners innately subscribe to the ethical principles of beneficence (doing good), nonmaleficence (doing no harm), and justice (fairness, equality). Specific areas within the codes may address these as well as other ethical principles.

Ethical codes are intended to specify distinct areas of values and standards of behavior to which practitioners should subscribe. They are intended as guides to the daily practice of specific disciplines. It should also be recognized that people can disagree in their interpretation of ethics and ethical codes.[4]

What, specifically, should an ethical code do? According to Helmicks, it should:

- Describe in practical terms the values held by the profession
- Impose obligations on professionals to accept both the values and the practices described in the code
- Hold professionals responsible for those obligations, with possible penalties for not conforming to the code

CODE OF ETHICS: SOCIETY OF NUCLEAR MEDICINE–TECHNOLOGISTS' SECTION

There are seven principles in this code. The preamble states:

> Nuclear medicine technologists, as members of the health care profession, must strive as individuals and as a group to maintain the highest ethical standards. The Principles listed below were adopted by the Technologists' Section of the Society of Nuclear Medicine at the 1985 Winter Meeting. They are not laws, but standards of conduct to be used as a quick guide by nuclear medicine technologists.

Principle 1

The nuclear medicine technologist should provide service with compassion and respect the rights of the patient.

This principle directly addresses beneficence as well as the relationship between patient and practitioner. Haas[6] has identified two primary models of relationship between patient and practitioner. The first is a Hippocratic (paternalistic) model which views the physician or health-care provider (the physician's extension) as the ultimate authority regarding decisions about the patient. The second is the contractual model, in which providers are expected to provide quality care, but the patient is at least an equal in the decision-making process. Although the first model is more convenient for the health-care provider, the second is more widely accepted today.

According to Mundy,[7] this principle indirectly addresses patient rights and autonomy, including the right to refuse examinations. She notes that if patients want to refuse an examination, it is the duty of the staff as well as the primary care physician to ensure that the patients have the information necessary to make an informed decision. If they still wish to refuse at that time, the medical imaging professional must respect that decision.

Principle 2

The nuclear medicine technologist should hold in strict confidence all privileged information concerning the patient.

Health-care professionals are expected to respect all individuals, and one of the most basic types of respect is respect of privacy. This code, unlike the ultrasound and radiologic technology codes discussed later in the chapter, fails to mention law. The legal status of technologists in the provision of medical information has not been firmly established. Although there are no confidentiality laws, such as those that cover the attorney-client relationship, there are constraints on divulging information. Obvious examples include patients who are a danger to themselves or others.

Principle 3

The nuclear medicine technologist should comply with the laws and regulations governing the practice of nuclear medicine.

Nuclear medicine is probably the most regulated of the medical imaging professions. Most of the regulations are designed to minimize the exposure of patients undergoing nuclear medicine procedures. Normally, law and ethics are separate considerations; this is one example in which law and ethics meet. Laws not specific to nuclear medicine are excluded. For example, although it is both morally and legally wrong for a nuclear medicine technologist to cheat on his or her income taxes, this action does not relate to the Code.

Principle 4

The nuclear medicine technologist should be responsible for competent performance of assigned duties.

Competence is a recognized concern in all the health professions.[8] One document that helps to define competence in nuclear medicine is the "Performance and Responsibility Guidelines for the Nuclear Medicine Technologist," developed by the Socio-Economic Affairs Committee of the Technologists' Section of the Society of Nuclear Medicine.[9]

Nuclear medicine is unique among imaging modalities in that unsealed radioactive isotopes or radiopharmaceuticals are used to image a patient. Working with unsealed radioactive sources requires certain competencies from the technologist. For example, cleaning up small radioactive spills (e.g., patient urine in some studies) from the work area will avoid contamination on or near a gamma camera. Such spills can create artifacts that could cause the physician to err in the interpretation of the study.

Principle 5

The nuclear medicine technologist should strive continuously to improve knowledge and skills.

Continuing education is one means of improving knowledge and skills. In many settings, nuclear medicine technologists must secure continuing education credits or "points" to maintain certification or licensure. However, the ethical professional should view continuing education as more than a search for mandatory points and strive to make that education relevant to his or her career. Improving knowledge logically includes being a member of professional medical groups and spending time in the medical library researching topics of interest.

In today's managed care and multiskilled environment, the medical imaging professional who is multiskilled and multicredentialed will not only be more employable, but will help the profession of nuclear medicine as well, by showing the value and adaptability of nuclear medicine.

Principle 6

The nuclear medicine technologist should not engage in fraud or deception.

Nuclear medicine is a highly regulated imaging modality, with federal, state, and local regulatory agencies requiring strict adherence to law. Although complacency may occur in maintaining the many regulations over time, poor record keeping is not acceptable and could be construed as deception. All regulations are made to protect the patient and the technologist. Therefore, when fraudulent actions do take place, technologists are placing themselves or their patients at more risk than is allowed by law. For example, it is rumored that some nuclear medicine technologists engage in a practice referred to as "juicing up a patient," in which the patient is given more of a radiopharmaceutical than is needed to complete the examination. Supposedly, extra radiopharmaceuticals are administered to make the examination proceed faster. The amount administered is often recorded as the lower, allowable amount. This is a clear case of fraud, if in fact it does occur.

Mundy[7] believes that this principle also relates to the process of informed consent, in that inaccurate information, coercion, or intimidation are not appropriate means of securing consent. For example, if a patient asks, "Will I receive radiation from this machine?" (referring to the gamma camera), and the technologist answers, "No," without explaining to the patient that the radiation has already been administered by injection of the isotope, this could be seen as deception. Similarly, telling a patient that a nuclear medicine scan "Is not like an x ray" might also be deception, since it tends to make the patient think no radiation is involved. The ethical principle of autonomy tells us that every individual has the right to determine his or her own destiny. Included within that right is the right to decide what type of medical care, procedure, and so forth is in the individual's best interest. The only way an individual can adequately determine what is best is to have enough knowledge about the treatment or procedure. When a medical imaging professional withholds information, does not give correct information, or simply does not provide enough information, the patient's autonomy is threatened.

Principle 7

The nuclear medicine technologist should be willing to assume responsibility to participate in activities that promote community and national response to health needs.

Any health-care worker should be willing to help in the event of a disaster, whether natural or an event like the Oklahoma City bombing. Skills such as starting an IV, taking a blood pressure, taking vital signs, or even skilled patient transportation may be needed in an emergency situation. For example, nuclear medicine technologists have the basic skills necessary to assist in helping decontaminate radiation accident victims and should be prepared to contribute those skills to society if needed.

Also, nuclear medicine technologists are expected to educate the public about radiation and its uses.[9] Both Jensen[10] and Wagner[11] note that nuclear medicine is an effective modality, but this fact is not often communicated to referring physicians or the general public. The need to communicate will increase, Jensen notes, with an increase in managed care, in which the bottom line is all-important. He notes, "If we are in nuclear medicine because we know it helps patients, don't we owe an education to those who don't know it?"[10]

CODE OF PROFESSIONAL CONDUCT FOR DIAGNOSTIC MEDICAL SONOGRAPHERS

There are five principles in this code. The preamble to the code states:

> The Code of Professional Conduct of the Society of Diagnostic Medical Sonographers is a statement of the high standards of conduct toward which sonographers are committed to strive. Sonographers, as members of a health care profession, acknowledge their responsibilities to their patients, to other health care professionals, and to each other.

Principle 1

Sonographers shall act in the best interests of the patient.

As in Principle 1 of the nuclear medicine code, this code recognizes the need for the practitioner to use beneficence as the guiding force behind clinical practice. Practitioners should realize that what they see as the "best outcome" may not be the best outcome for the patient; medical ethicists have described this as a conflict between the ethical principles of autonomy and beneficence.[6,12]

Medical imaging professionals are educated to believe that certain procedures are beneficial to the patient. In our clinical experience, seeing a "good outcome" tends to confirm these views. However, only the patient can decide what is best based on a personal value assessment of the situation. Brian Clark's play *Whose Life Is It Anyway?*, in which a paralyzed patient wants to end his life, is an excellent example of this conflict.[13,14] Medical imaging professionals must always strive to "do good" while realizing that, in the end, only patients can define what is good for them according to parameters over which only they have control (autonomy).

Principle 2

Sonographers shall provide sonographic services with compassion, respect for human dignity, honesty, and integrity.

What distinguishes a profession from a trade? According to Stromberg,[15] although a tradesperson respects the basic rights of an individual, a profit motive is always the guiding principle. However, professionals hold themselves to higher standards, primarily in the area of service to others. This principle may take on added importance for sonographers in the newly forming managed care environment, in which profit motives may take precedence over service.

Principle 3

Sonographers shall respect the patient's right to privacy, safeguarding confidential information within the constraints of the law.

Confidentiality is a basic right based on respect for people. All professionals should know the circumstances in which they should not reveal information about a patient, as well as the circumstances in which they should.

> **DISCUSSION QUESTION**
> A sonographer knows a patient very well. The patient has a chronic disease that is rather debilitating, but which allows mostly normal function. One day this patient comes in for an examination, appearing rather despondent. She talks vaguely about euthanasia and the "courage of some people to end it all when life is no longer worth living." Should this information be kept confidential? How should the sonographer respond?

Principle 4

Sonographers shall maintain competence in their field.

Since sonographers often engage in some basic screening or diagnosis, it is very important that they develop these skills and maintain them based on current technology and practice standards. Since there are still a limited number of ultrasound programs in this country, it may be difficult for a practitioner to find a local program. In such cases, sonographers are expected to work together to develop an organization such as a branch of the SDMS for the continuing education needs of sonographers in the area. It should be remembered that continuing education is just one part of a total equation (along with skills development and maintenance) to bring about continuing competence.

Principle 5

Sonographers shall assume responsibility for their actions.

Professionals accept responsibility for their actions. They do not hide behind other professionals, such as physicians or the institution. Again, since sonographers often perform some basic screening or diagnosis, they should accept the responsibility for doing so. This may increase their professional liability, but individuals assuming a role need to accept responsibility for that role.

AMERICAN SOCIETY OF RADIOLOGIC TECHNOLOGISTS—CODE OF ETHICS

The Code of Ethics of the ASRT (listed as one portion of the American Registry of Radiologic Technologists [ARRT] Standards of Ethics) enumerates aspirational goals designed to foster a high level of ethical conduct for radiologic science professionals. The ARRT also has enforceable Rules of Ethics contained with the Standards.

The April 1996 ARRT Annual Report to Registered Technologists provides information regarding proposed revisions to the Standards of Ethics. These revisions are intended to clearly define violations of the Rules of Ethics contained within the document. Also in the Annual Report, for the first time, is a list of individuals whose ARRT certification was revoked by the Ethics Committee for conduct deemed in violation of the ARRT Standards of Ethics between October of 1993 and October of 1995. The names of 53 individuals appeared along with their birth date, ARRT certification number, and city and state of residence. The age range for the individuals was 25 to 52 years. The state having the most revocations was Texas, with five. New Jersey, Illinois, and California followed with four each. Technologists in 23 states had ARRT certification revocations.

Reaction to the publication of the names by individuals contacted by the authors has been mixed. Some feel that since the revocation of the certification was for violation of ethical standards, the publication of names and other information is a service to the public. By publishing the names, birth dates, certificate numbers, and city and state of residence, these individuals are less likely to be hired into positions in which good moral character is required. Others feel that the publication of such data actually violated the medical imaging professional's right to privacy.

While the ASRT Code of Ethics is only a small portion of the ARRT Standards of Ethics, it provides the medical imaging professional with rules by which to practice.

Principle 1

The Radiologic Technologist conducts himself/herself in a professional manner, responds to patient needs, and supports colleagues and associates in providing quality patient care.

This principle establishes the radiologic science technologist as a professional health-care worker. A professional is distinguished from a paraprofessional by accepting responsibility for actions, knowing why things are done, and being capable of independent thought and judgment.

This principle makes the radiologic technologist responsible for responding to patients' needs; thus, he or she cannot be seen as a mere "film-shooter." The responsibilities of the profession include responding to physical and emotional needs of all types of patients. It also makes the radiologic science professional a colleague of all professional health-care workers, with appropriate rights and responsibilities. These responsibilities adhere to the ethical principle of fidelity (faithfulness).

Principle 2

The Radiologic Technologist acts to advance the principal objective of the profession to provide services to humanity with full respect for the dignity of mankind.

This principle recognizes that the radiologic technologist is an individual with education appropriate to understanding human needs. It also instructs the radiologic technologist to place the dignity of patients first and foremost in his or her mind. All patients deserve to be thought of as individuals and treated with dignity. This principle establishes the basic concept of beneficence found in all health-care ethical codes.

Principle 3

The Radiologic Technologist delivers patient care and service unrestricted by concerns of personal attributes or the nature of the disease or illness, and without discrimination, regardless of sex, race, creed, religion, or socioeconomic status.

This principle instructs the radiologic technologist not to allow personal attributes, the nature of the illness, or discrimination to influence care. Principles 2 and 3 are similar in terms of intent. Can a radiologic technologist refuse to care for patients with AIDS from an ethical standpoint? No. Although some institutions allow workers to refuse to treat certain kinds of patients, and some ethicists believe that personal freedom should allow individuals to refuse to care for certain patients, a radiologic technologist would be violating Principle 3 of the code by refusing to care for a patient with AIDS. Radiologic technologists are expected to know and use measures such as universal precautions in handling all patients so as not to discriminate against those with certain transmittable disorders. The paternalistic role of medical imaging professionals and other health-care providers dictates that they do what is best for the patient regardless of race, age, socioeconomic attributes, and so on. An old medical aphorism instructs professionals to "hate the disease, not the patient that has the disease."

Principle 4

The Radiologic Technologist practices technology founded upon theoretical knowledge and concepts, utilizes equipment and accessories consistent with the purpose for which they have been designed, and employs procedures and techniques appropriately.

This principle ensures that radiologic technologists use only accepted theory and concepts in the production of diagnostic images or in administering therapy. It also ensures that they will use equipment only as designed, and instructs them to know accepted procedures and techniques. As Warner[16] stated about an earlier version of this principle:

> Equipment can be designed, manufactured, and tested to meet rigid compliance standards. But it is the use of that equipment on a daily basis by the technologist that may or may not lack scientific basis. Technique charts, quality assurance programs, repeat analysis and gonadal shielding all have a scientific framework, but are they used consistently by the technologist?

This principle also has particular relevance to educators in medical imaging. It is their direct responsibility to introduce the student to theories and facts surrounding the profession so that practitioners possess the knowledge to fulfill the principle.

Principle 5

The Radiologic Technologist assesses situations, exercises care, discretion and judgment, assumes responsibility for professional decisions, and acts in the best interest of the patient.

This principle, which is similar to Principle 1, makes the radiologic technologist responsible for assessing the needs of patients and situations and for decisions made. It also indicates that the best interest of the patient (beneficence) is of the utmost importance in treating patients.

Principle 6

The Radiologic Technologist acts as an agent through observation and communication to obtain pertinent information for the physician to aid in the diagnosis and treatment management of the patient, and recognizes that interpretation and diagnosis are outside the scope of practice for the profession.

This principle indicates that the radiologic technologist has a role as an extension of the physician in improving patient care. This recognition is unique to this code.

This principle also recognizes that radiologic technologists will not provide interpretation and diagnosis; however, it does not establish them as incapable of making a diagnosis. A radiologic technologist, for example, must be able to make some basic assessment of a radiograph to ensure that it is of diagnostic quality, but the technologist may not provide diagnosis from a film to patients or other health professionals, except as indicated (i.e., physician's orders).

> **DISCUSSION QUESTION**
> Consider the following scenario. You have done everything you can to convince Ms. Jones, an elderly patient, of the need for an x ray of her hip. Her leg has the outward sign of a fractured hip; however, she is very anxious and fearful of the examination. You contact the radiologist, who goes into the room to talk with the patient. When he leaves the room, he says to you, "Do it anyway. I'll take the responsibility." What are the ethical responsibilities here? Are there any ethical principles in the ASRT Code of Ethics that are in conflict? What do you do?

Principle 7

The Radiologic Technologist utilizes equipment and accessories, employs techniques and procedures, performs services in accordance with an accepted standard of practice, and demonstrates expertise in limiting the radiation exposure to the patient, self, and other members of the health care team.

This principle requires that the radiologic technologist understand the scope of practice of the profession, and it makes radiation protection a primary role of the technologist, equal to producing diagnostic films and providing therapy and patient care.

Principle 8

The Radiologic Technologist practices ethical conduct appropriate to the profession, and protects the patient's right to quality radiologic technology care.

This principle reinforces the need for ethical conduct. Ethics is *not* simply good manners. It is a moral way of thinking and acting. Principle 8 also reinforces (for the third time) the right of the patient to quality care.

Principle 9

The Radiologic Technologist respects confidences entrusted in the course of professional practice, protects the patient's right to privacy, and reveals confidential information only as required by law or to protect the welfare of the individuals or the community.

This principle establishes confidentiality as part of the radiologic technologist's practice. It allows confidentiality to be breached only under conditions of law or extreme need. Read back through the examples provided for nuclear medicine and sonography if it is still unclear when information should and should not be revealed. Realize also that this is learned well only through years of clinical experience.

Annas[17] notes that beyond the release of information, the patient also has the following privacy rights:

- To refuse to see any visitors
- To refuse to see anyone not officially connected with the hospital
- To refuse to see anyone not involved in his or her care or treatment, including social workers or chaplains
- To wear personal nightclothes (unless medically contraindicated) and religious medallions
- To refuse to have a person of the opposite sex present when disrobing
- To remain disrobed only long enough for medical procedures
- To insist on a room transfer if a roommate is disturbing him or her

Principle 10

The Radiologic Technologist continually strives to improve knowledge and skills by participating in educational and professional activities, sharing knowledge with colleagues and investigating new and innovative aspects of professional practice. One means available to improve knowledge and skills is through professional continuing education.

This principle requires a radiologic technologist to remain up to date in

TABLE 3–1
SIMILARITIES AMONG THE PROFESSIONAL CODES

Beneficence	Confidentiality	Competency and Continued Education	Patient Rights
SNM–TS 1	SNM–TS 2	SNM–TS 4	SNM–TS 1
SDMS 1	SDMS 3	SNM–TS 5	ASRT 2
ASRT 5	ASRT 9	SDMS 4	ASRT 3
		ASRT 4	ASRT 8
		ASRT 7	SDMS 2
		ASRT 10	

Practitioner Autonomy	Law	Physician's Agent or Assistant	Public Education
SDMS 5	SNM–TS 3	ASRT 6	SNM–TS 7
ASRT 1	SNM–TS 6		
ASRT 5	SDMS 3		
	ASRT 9		
	(Last two only in		
	tandem with		
	confidentiality)		

The number following each abbreviation indicates the numbered principle of each code.
SNM–TS = Society of Nuclear Medicine–Technologists' Section; SDMS = Society of Diagnostic Medical Sonographers; ASRT = American Society of Radiologic Technologists.

terms of knowledge and to increase that knowledge base in the radiologic sciences. Few technologists publish in the radiologic sciences; however, sharing knowledge is an ethical imperative. Even staff medical imaging professionals can conduct research at the clinical level, and they are obligated to share that research with colleagues through in-service presentations, presentations at staff meetings, or through peer-reviewed publications. Any medical imaging professional who discovers a new or better way of doing things should find a means to share that with the community of practitioners and scholars.

SIMILARITIES AMONG THE THREE PROFESSIONAL CODES

Understanding what the three codes of ethics have in common helps us to understand the basic underpinnings of ethical codes. Also, since many medical imaging professionals operate under multiple codes (e.g. a practitioner may be a sonographer and radiologic technologist or nuclear medicine technologist), it is important to have a clear view of the ethical expectations of the profession as a whole.

Table 3–1 summarizes the commonalities of the codes. All three codes call directly for beneficence, confidentiality, competency, recognition of patient's rights (especially patient advocacy), and adherence to law. Law is mentioned in the ASRT and Sonographer codes only in relation to confidentiality. The Nuclear Medicine code calls for public education, and the ASRT asserts the role of the radiologic technologist as an assistant to the physician.

The ASRT code appears to be the most comprehensive. However, many of the statements also cover multiple roles (see, for example, principle 5, which covers patient assessment and autonomy), which could lead to a lack of clarity in interpretation by practitioners, or by an agency enforcing the code, such as the ARRT.

WHISTLEBLOWING

One of the most complex ethical dilemmas for health-care professionals is whistleblowing, which may be considered an extension of patient advocacy.[18] Whistleblowing is "an attempt on the part of someone in an organization to disclose or call attention to some perceived wrongdoing in the organization."[19] It can be subdivided into internal whistleblowing, which is informing higher management about problems by going over the boss's head, or external whistleblowing, which is informing an outside body or person, such as a regulatory agency or a newspaper reporter.

In many cases, the whistleblower is protected legally.[20] The First Amendment to the U.S. Constitution protects freedom of speech. Public sector employees are protected by the Civil Service Reform Act of 1979, The Whistleblower Protection Act of 1969, the Department of Defense Authorization Act, and in some cases, state statutes. Private-sector employees may be covered by the Energy Reorganization Act, the Federal Mine Safety and Health Act, the Occupational Safety and Health Act (OSHA), or a number of other federal acts.

For example, the Nuclear Regulatory Commission (NRC) has cited and fined a hospital for not allowing an employee to discuss safety concerns with the NRC.[21] The employee's supervisor issued a letter to the hospital's radiology chair that stated displeasure with her "bad-mouthing" the department following an NRC inspection. The NRC found that such actions could create what is commonly called a "chilling effect," which would discourage employees from bringing information to the NRC about possible regulatory violations.

An earlier case (*Richter v. Ellis Fischel State Cancer Center*)[22] involved a radiation safety officer who discovered that four radioactive iridium seeds implanted in a cancer patient had not been removed before her dismissal from the hospital. After a report to the NRC, a number of events occurred that eventually resulted in Richter's dismissal. Richter successfully sued for discrimination.

Ethically, three questions should be considered before whistleblowing[19]:

1. How serious is the unethical or illegal behavior? If there is an in-

creased ability to cause harm or a flagrant violation of basic rights, the need to report increases.
2. What is the strength of the evidence? The facts must be clear, both to prove the case and to prevent possible damage to a professional reputation based on unsubstantiated evidence.
3. What are the normal channels for resolving the issue? Have they been attempted? It is logical to exhaust normal reporting options unless they are unviable (e.g., the person you would report the violation to is the one committing the violation), and it is usually best to attempt internal whistle-blowing before external options, given certain constraints.

The whistleblower must also consider the negative outcomes of whistleblowing, both to the organization and to him or herself. Studies have shown a number of reprisals are directed at whistleblowers, including reassignment or dismissal, blacklisting, and physical violence.[23] One study showed that 17% of whistleblowers had lost their homes, 10% had attempted suicide, and 8% had gone bankrupt.[18] Fellow employees may shun the whistleblower.[23,24] Legal remedies are rarely adequate and may take years to resolve after the event occurred.[25] Thus, the potential whistleblower may be prone to "swallow the whistle" rather than blow it.[26]

However, as Gillet notes, the moral imperative in health care makes the right to speak out against wrongdoing of particular importance.[27] Society should support that right if at all possible in order to protect patients from harm. Medical imaging professionals must also recognize that their role as patient advocates makes whistleblowing one of their primary ethical duties.

DISCUSSION QUESTION
You are the quality assurance technologist in a small community hospital. You have informed the chief technologist three times now that the x-ray beam/light beam congruence greatly exceeds acceptable standards. Finally, he says, "Look, the technologists know how to adapt to it, so fixing it would just confuse them." How do you address this?

CONCLUSION

All medical imaging professionals should be familiar with the demands of the ethical code for their specialty. They should let these codes guide their professional practice. The guidelines in these codes are designed to protect the patient and society and to promote the profession of medical imaging in a positive manner.

REFERENCES

 1. Singarella, R, and Salladay, S: Ethical considerations for the biomedical communications professional. Journal of Biocommunications 1:10, 1981.
 2. Craig, M: Introduction to Ultrasonography and Patient Care. Philadelphia, WB Saunders, 1994.
 3. Dowd, SB: Patient Consent. Albuquerque, NM, American Society of Radiologic Technologists, 1994.
 4. Golden, DG: Medical ethics courses for student technologists. Radiologic Technology 62(6):452–459, 1991.
 5. Helmick, JW: Ethics and the profession of audiology. Seminars in Hearing 15:190–197, 1994.
 6. Haas, J: Ethical considerations of goal setting for patient care in rehabilitation medicine. American Journal of Physical Medicine and Rehabilitation 72:228–232, 1993.
 7. Mundy, WM: Ethical practice in nuclear medicine technology. Journal of Nuclear Medicine Technology 19:44–49, 1991.
 8. Evert, MM: Competency: Ethical issues and dilemmas. The American Journal of Occupational Therapy 47:487–489, 1993.
 9. Higgins, D, Hall, A, Clarke, M, et al: Performance and responsibility guidelines for the nuclear medicine technologist. Journal of Nuclear Medicine Technology 22:255–260, 1994.
10. Jensen, DG: Communicating the value of nuclear medicine in a changing health care environment. Journal of Nuclear Medicine Technology 23:93–98, 1995.
11. Wagner, H: Newsline. Journal of Nuclear Medicine Technology 35:26N, 1994.
12. Veatch, RM: A Theory of Medical Ethics. New York, Basic Books, 1981.
13. Clark, B. Whose Life Is It Anyway? New York, Avon, 1978.
14. Meier, RH, and Purtilo, RB: Ethical issues and the patient-provider relationship. American Journal of Physical Medicine and Rehabilitation 73:365–366, 1994.
15. Stromberg, CD: Key legal issues in professional ethics. In Goldsmith, SC, and Ciuccio, JH (eds): Reflections on Ethics. Washington, DC, American Speech-Language-Hearing Association, 1990.
16. Warner, SB: Code of ethics: Professional and legal implications. Radiologic Technology 52(5):485–494, 1981.
17. Annas, GJ: The Rights of Patients, ed 2. Carbondale, Ill, Southern Illinois University Press.
18. O'Connor, T: Whistling up a storm. Nursing New Zealand 2(2):2, 1994.
19. Weber, LJ, and Bissell, MG: Whistleblowing. Clinical Laboratory Management Review 8:356, 358–359, 1994.
20. Fenton, RD: Whistleblower protection. In Obergfell, AM (ed): Law and Ethics in Diagnostic Imaging and Therapeutic Radiology. Philadelphia, WB Saunders, 1995:151–158.
21. Hospital Allegedly Discriminated Against Oncology Tech. Radiology & Imaging Letter 15(20):157, 1995.
22. Richter v. Ellis Fischel State Cancer Center (Missouri 1981).
23. Westin, AF: Whistleblowing! New York, McGraw-Hill, 1981.
24. Kiely, MA, and Kiely, DC: Whistleblowing: disclosure and its consequences for the professional nurse and management. Nursing Management 18(5):41–45, 1987.
25. Carr, A: Should a nurse report a nurse? Nursing Mirror 156(12):26, 1983.
25. Feliu, A: The role of the law in protecting scientific and technical dissent. Presented at the American Association for the Advancement of Science Annual Meeting, New York, May 1984.
26. Banja, JD: Whistleblowing in physical therapy. Physical Therapy 65:1683–1686, 1985.
27. Gillet, G: The right to speak out. Hospimedica 1991 (October), p 23.

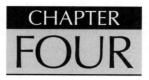

CHAPTER FOUR

Ethical Problem-Solving Techniques

Bettye G. Wilson, MEd, RT(R)(CT), RDMS

This chapter describes the types of ethical problems likely to be encountered by medical imaging professionals. Examples of each type are provided to assist the student in solving ethical problems. A general outline for solving complex ethical problems is included, as well as a model step-by-step process for making ethical decisions.

OBJECTIVES

At the end of this chapter, the reader will be able to:

- List the four types of ethical problems
- Recognize the specific type of ethical problem when provided with the parameters associated with that type of problem
- Provide examples for each type of ethical problem discussed in the chapter
- List and define the seven universal ethical principles
- Describe the general decision-making techniques for solving complex ethical problems
- Apply the step-by-step process of ethical problem-solving presented in this chapter

ETHICAL SCENARIO

You have just completed an acute abdomen series on Mrs. Andrews. While waiting for her radiographs to be developed, you engage her in conversation. She tells you that you have been her radiographer before and she appreciates your professionalism. She also tells you that she has had abdominal surgery in the last few days and actually feels worse than she did before that. She is now experiencing acute abdominal pain and distension and has an elevated temperature. She asks you if you are familiar with the work of her surgeon, Dr. Awe. Is he a good surgeon? Are his patients prone to postsurgical infections? She then asks, you think jokingly, if he has ever been known to leave surgical apparatus in his patients. You tell her that you'll answer her questions immediately after you check the quality of her radiographs.

When you view Mrs. Andrews' radiographs, you note what appear to be a surgical hemostat and a sponge on her films. You immediately check Mrs. Andrews for the presence of these items extrinsically. You find nothing. You then show the films to the radiologist. She confirms the presence of surgical items and asks you to make additional abdominal radiographs in lateral projection.

What do you tell Mrs. Andrews about the need for additional radiographs? How do you answer, or should you answer, the questions she asked before your discovery?

ETHICAL PROBLEMS

The preceding scenario poses an ethical problem that can arise in professional practice when one cares about doing a better-than-average job.[1] As discussed in Chapter Two, personal behaviors are based on our value system. Problems may be encountered when differing value systems conflict.[2] Inevitably, ethical problems must be solved by placing one set of values above others.[3] As the field of medicine continues to grow in terms of new discoveries and technological advancements, more ethical problems will be created for which solutions will not be easily found.[4] Indeed, ethical problems arise when a situation creates conflict between two or more moral norms or principles. According to Purtilo,[5] not all ethical problems are equal. She has identified four types of ethical problems:

1. Ethical dilemmas
2. Ethical dilemmas of justice
3. Ethical distress
4. Locus of authority issues

Ethical Dilemmas

Ethical dilemmas are created when one is faced with a situation in which there is actually more than one ethical course of action. However, in taking one course, you are precluded from taking the other. In other words, a choice must be made between two ethical actions.

To facilitate a better understanding of ethical dilemmas, return to the ethical scenario presented at the beginning of this chapter. If you as the radiographer hold the ethical principle of beneficence (performing acts or actions beneficial to others) as one of your moral values, and further subscribe to the duty-based principle of veracity (truth telling) while also holding a belief that you have a moral obligation to your facility, this scenario may pose an ethical dilemma.

There are at least two possible courses of action that the radiographer in the scenario could pursue. First, he or she could answer Mrs. Andrews' questions honestly, even telling her that Dr. Awe has left surgical apparatus inside patients, since radiographs of several of his previous patients have revealed the presence of such apparatus. This course of action would be in keeping with beneficence by providing information that may benefit Mrs. Andrews in her quest to understand why, after surgery, she feels much worse than she did preoperatively. Also, by providing factual information to Mrs. Andrews in response to her questions concerning Dr. Awe, the radiographer would be upholding the principle of veracity. As a second course of action, however, the radiographer could perceive the principle of beneficence in a different light by finding it more beneficial not to disclose knowledge of the situation. In essence, he or she would place beneficence over veracity in this case. This may be primarily a response to the need for the radiographer to uphold a moral obligation to the facility of employment, which includes doing nothing to cast the employees of the facility in a negative light. It is obvious that both of these courses of action cannot be followed. A choice must be made and adhered to. This is an ethical dilemma.

> **DISCUSSION QUESTION**
> Review the ethical scenario presented at the beginning of the chapter again. Can you find at least two other courses of action the radiographer could pursue? List the pros and cons of pursuing each of the possible choices. How does one choice preclude the radiographer from following the other?

Ethical Dilemmas of Justice

Ethical dilemmas of justice are problems that arise in association with the distribution of benefits and burdens on a societal basis. In health care, this involves the allocation of scarce resources. The term "distributive justice" is often used, although other terms, such as "compensatory," "corrective," and "retributive," may also be used. Health care in the United States is distributed at two levels, macroallocation and microallocation. According to *Webster's New World Dictionary,*[7] the term "allocate" means to set apart for a specific purpose or to distribute in shares or according to a plan. The term "macroallocation" is used to describe widespread or long-term distribution of health care. It is usually seen as the job of Congress, state legislatures, insurance companies, health organizations, and private foundations to determine macroallocation in health care. Microallocation of health care goods and services, in contrast, is seen as a more personal determination of who will receive scarce resources at the local level.[8]

DISCUSSION QUESTION

Can you think of health-care distribution issues that fall under the umbrella of macroallocation? Under microallocation?

In the medical imaging profession, ethical dilemmas of justice occur at the microallocation level and usually involve such questions as who will receive the benefit of advanced imaging technology, such as computed tomography (CT), magnetic resonance (MR), and positron emission tomography (PET); or how, in this time of health-care manpower cutbacks, to prioritize the delivery of services.

DISCUSSION QUESTION

Most medical facilities triage emergency department patients in that they sort or group them based on the severity of the injury or illness. Is triage a means of solving ethical dilemmas of justice? Can you think of other situations directly applicable to imaging practice?

Ethical Distress

Ethical distress is created when there is an obvious correct solution to an ethical problem but institutional constraints prohibit the correct solution from being applied.[5] For example, working as a trauma radiographer in a large emergency department, you notice that people who arrive in respiratory arrest are placed on mechanical ventilation before a complete assessment of their condition is made. More times than not, these patients are later found to have experienced oxygen deprivation for too long, and days later they are declared clinically dead. The next of kin are then asked for permission to disconnect the ventilator, which creates a serious ethical problem for the family. You know that the solution to this problem is to have all patients who arrive in respiratory arrest evaluated as to the extent of the problem causing the arrest and the length of time the patient experienced arrest without the benefit of oxygen. In this way, families of individuals who basically have no hope of recovery could be spared having to make a decision concerning what they may believe is the life or death of their loved one.

You and others at your facility agree that this is the best course of action; however, institutional policy requires that anyone entering the emergency department in respiratory arrest be immediately placed on a ventilator and every attempt made to save that person's life. Hospital administration and others on the medical staff consider this a wonderful policy in and of itself. However, it may create problems for the families of those who are too critical to be saved and must then be removed from the ventilator.

DISCUSSION QUESTION
What do you think about the emergency department situation just presented? Do you agree that decisions concerning the removal of mechanical ventilators from brain-dead individuals create ethical distress for the family of the patient? Why or why not? Can you think of other examples of ethical distress that you have encountered in practice, read about, or heard about?

Locus of Authority Issues

Locus of authority issues occur when there are questions regarding who is responsible or under whose authority something falls. Also, confusion may exist as to who has the ultimate decision-making power in a given situation. You may have sensed a locus of authority issue lurking in the ethical scenario presented at the beginning of the chapter. Whose responsibility is it to inform Mrs. Andrews as to the nature of her postsurgical abdominal problems? Does it fall within the sphere of duty of the radiographer, radiologist, attending physician, nurse, surgeon, or some administrative authority?

Locus of authority issues may sometimes be resolved by simply following the chain of command in reporting the issue. Problems may be encountered when those in authority will not assume responsibility for making a decision or taking action to solve a problem. Generally speaking, however, most people in authority willingly accept their responsibilities in making decisions and taking charge of situations.

DISCUSSION QUESTION

Do you know to whom you should report the following situations at your institution?

1. Suspected nonaccidental trauma (child abuse)
2. Patient falls
3. Administration of incorrect medication
4. Patient compliments or criticisms regarding care in the department

PROBLEM SOLVING

Ethical problems of differing scopes and magnitudes will be encountered throughout our lives. The four types of ethical problems just discussed are the most common. They may exist alone or in combination. They may be simple or complex. It is generally not known in advance what type or types of ethical problems will be encountered. However, what can be known in advance is what values, ethical codes, principles, techniques, and steps may be applied to solve a problem. Finding solutions to ethical problems in the medical imaging field requires:

- Having a clear understanding of your own personal values (see Chap. Two)
- Understanding the professional code of ethics and/or conduct under which your practice falls (see Chap. Three)
- Applying the seven principles of biomedical ethics, to be discussed next
- Employing effective decision-making techniques
- Using a step-by-step approach in making ethical decisions

The Seven Principles of Biomedical Ethics

The principles of medical ethics provide those of us practicing in the healing arts and sciences with a common morality.[9] These same principles provide the foundation for the codes of ethics and conduct upon which those in all spheres of medicine base their practice. It seems that these principles did not come about in unison, but have been amassed over time. To date, these seven have been identified:

1. Autonomy
2. Beneficence
3. Confidentiality
4. Justice
5. Nonmaleficence

6. Role fidelity
7. Veracity[8]

At first glance, these ethical principles may not seem related. On closer examination, however, a common thread may be found—all may be viewed as concepts of duty or obligation. As described in Chapter One, deontology is the duty-based ethical theory under which those in the medical professions practice. These duty-based ethical principles, which are essential to ethical decision making, were defined in Chapter One.

DISCUSSION QUESTION
Referring to the list of the seven ethical principles and to their respective meanings in Chapter One, can you think of everyday work situations in which you employ each of these principles? Describe them.

Decision-Making Techniques for Solving Complex Problems

Loewy[10] has asserted that analyzing and ultimately finding solutions to ethical problems is not that fundamentally different from solving problems in other fields. He and other authors agree that sorting out ethical problems requires specific analysis and thought. Guy[11] goes a step further by proclaiming that decision making in solving ethical problems should maximize particular values and should occur in ordered steps. She presents the following 10 steps for solving complex problems:

1. Define the problem.
2. Identify the goal to be achieved.
3. Specify all dimensions of the problem.
4. List all possible solutions to each dimension.
5. Evaluate alternative solutions to each dimension regarding the likelihood of each to maximize the important values at stake.
6. Eliminate alternatives that are too costly, not feasible, or maximize the wrong values when combined with other dimensions.
7. Rank the alternatives to each dimension according to which are most likely to maximize the most important values.
8. Select the alternative to each dimension that is most likely to work in the context of the problem while maximizing the important value at stake.
9. Combine the top-ranking alternatives for each dimension of the problem in order to develop a solution to the problem as a whole.
10. Make a commitment to the choice and implement it.

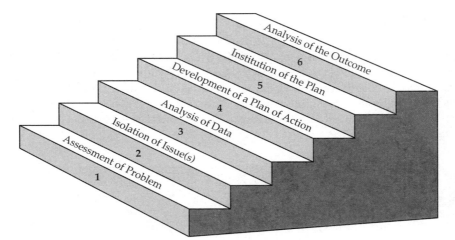

FIGURE 4–1. The Dowd model for ethical decision making.

Step-by-Step Approach to Ethical Decision Making

Society is asking for greater accountability from all professionals.[12] Hence, the greater need for education and training in resolving ethical problems in the workplace. In the allied health sciences, authors like Patterson and Vitello,[12] Golden,[13] Purtilo,[5] and Dowd[14] have presented simple step-by-step processes to assist in ethical decision making. The Dowd Model specifically addresses ethical problem solving as it relates to those in the medical imaging profession. It consists of six steps (Figure 4–1).

Step 1—Assessment of the Problem

This requires a determination as to which type of ethical problem is occurring (ethical dilemma, ethical dilemma of justice, ethical distress, or locus of authority issue).

Step 2—Isolation of the Issues

At this point, issues that are significant to the situation must be separated from those that are insignificant. A determination as to what values should be maximized should also be made. Consideration must be given as to which of the ethical principles are involved, which patient rights are being compromised, if any, and which principle or area of your professional code of ethics or conduct covers your behavior in situations of this type.

Step 3—Analysis of the Data

In this step, all pertinent information should be separated from pure conjecture. Only facts as they relate to the problem should be examined; all other issues should be deleted. List the facts and assign them under headings such as, but not limited to, the following:

- Ethical value promoted or compromised
- Rights of the patient violated or supported
- Your particular medical imaging professional code of ethics or conduct violated or supported
- Institutional policies and/or procedures upheld or desecrated

Step 4–Development of a Plan of Action

In this step, a decision should be made as to what options are available to solve the problem. Remember, you can only do one thing at a time, so a choice must be made. It should, of course, be the best ethically, from all the available alternatives.

Step 5—Institution of the Plan

At this step, proceed with your solution. Go ahead and do it. Hopefully, you have made the correct decision based on the due process provided in steps 1 through 5.

Step 6—Analysis of the Outcome

Did the plan work to your satisfaction? Were you satisfied with the outcome? Did others involved benefit from your plan? If this same situation, or one similar, occurs again, would you follow the same plan or find another solution?

CONCLUSION

Ethical problems in our personal life and professional practice occur more frequently than any of us desire. Ethical concerns cause us to undergo cognitive dissonance, a state in which our minds experience discord in trying to determine which of our ethical values, beliefs, theories, and so on are to be explored, evaluated, or upheld, and why this particular situation creates such problems for us.

It is probably easier to solve personal ethical problems than those of a professional nature. Professional ethical problems and their solutions are more taxing in that they require not only the examination of our personal value system, but also consideration of the professional codes of conduct under which we practice, the rights of the patients, and institutional policies and procedures. The ethical decision-making process, not withstanding, requires an orderly systematic approach as described in this chapter. Remember, ethical decision making or problem solving is an educational experience. Each problem, once solved, provides you with a learning experience that may be beneficial in approaching similar problems in the future.

REFERENCES

1. Monagle, JF, and Thomasma, DC: Medical Ethics A Guide for Health Professionals. Rockville, MD, Aspen, 1988.
2. Garlikov, R: A Virtue is a virtue, right? Not necessarily. The Birmingham News, Review and Comment Section, Sunday, September 11, 1994.
3. Bingold, JM, Malchoid, LR, and Terry, JS: Ethical dilemmas in the laboratory: The not-so-distant patient. Clinical Laboratory Science 1(4), 1988.
4. Lankard, BA: Resolving Ethical Dilemmas in the Workplace: A New Focus for Career Development. ERIC, Clearinghouse on Adult, Career, and Vocational Education. Digest No. 112, 1991, Ohio State University, 1991.
5. Purtilo, RB: Ethical Dimensions in the Health Professions, ed 2. Philadelphia, WB Saunders, 1993.
6. English, DC: Bioethics: A Clinical Guide for Medical Students. New York, Norton Medical Books, 1994.
7. Webster's New World Dictionary, ed 2. New York, Simon & Schuster, 1982.
8. Edge, RS, and Groves, JR: The Ethics of Health Care. Albany, Delmar, 1994.
9. Beauchamp, TL, and Childress, JF: Principles of Biomedical Ethics, ed 4. New York, Oxford Unversity Press, 1994.
10. Loewy, EH: Textbook of Medical Ethics. New York, Plenum Medical Book Company, 1989.
11. Guy, ME: Ethical Decision Making in Everyday Work Situations. New York, Quorum, 1990.
12. Patterson, SM, and Vitello, EM: Ethics in health education: The need to include a model course in professional preparation programs. Journal of Health Education (4):239–243, 1993.
13. Golden, DG: Medical ethics courses for student technologist. Radiologic Technology (6):452–457, 1991.
14. Dowd, SB: Ethical Decision Making [Computer Program]. Edwardsville, KS, Educational Softward Concepts, Inc., 1994.

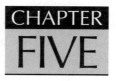

CHAPTER FIVE

Patient Consent

Steven B. Dowd, EdD, ARRT(R)

This chapter considers legal and ethical aspects of consent. Definitions of consent are sometimes confusing, so these are stressed, as are recent examinations of the use of agents (such as nurses and allied health professionals) in securing consent. Radiation experiments conducted in the 1940s through the 1960s are also discussed as they relate to historical views of consent and how this concept has changed over time.

OBJECTIVES
At the end of this chapter, the reader will be able to:
- Discuss the three aspects of consent
- List legal cases that relate to consent
- Explain the historical development of consent
- Give appropriate definitions of the various types of consent
- Describe the role of the medical imaging professional in securing consent

DEFINITION OF CONSENT

Patient consent is based on the principle of autonomy, which holds, in the medical setting, that adults are allowed to decide for themselves the care they feel is appropriate. A person in his or her right mind is able to determine whether a procedure is to be performed. Consent gives the health-care professional the right to touch and treat the patient.

51

There are three important aspects of consent:

1. **Communication**—a health-care professional (primarily the physician, although agents may also be appropriate) must tell the patient what he or she needs to know to decide what is the best course of treatment. In many cases, the health-care professional is serving as an educator to the patient to help him or her make effective decisions.
2. **Law**—patients have legal rights in the consent process established through guidelines and court cases.
3. **Ethics**—concepts such as beneficence (providing what the health-care professional sees as the "best" level of care) may conflict with patient autonomy (patients should be allowed to make even "bad" decisions, so long as they have all the information).

Consent exists, as do many concepts, on a continuum. Many procedures require only that the patient verbally, or by action, agree to have a procedure performed. This is called "simple consent," supposes no knowledge of the procedure, and simply involves obtaining a patient's permission to perform a procedure. It is further divided into express and implied consent. Express consent occurs when a patient climbs onto a table and allows an examination to be performed. Implied consent occurs in emergency situations, when the patient cannot decide, with a reasonable-person standard most often used. Legal difficulties can occur when simple consent is withdrawn by the patient; when it is exceeded, that is, when simple consent for one procedure is taken to be inclusive of others; or when this consent is overextended through consultation with other physicians or health-care providers.

Informed consent is a procedure whereby patients may agree to medical intervention or refuse it based on information provided by a health-care professional regarding the nature and possible consequences of the intervention. Providing this information is usually considered a duty of the physician, and he or she will probably remain ultimately responsible under the doctrine of respondeat superior (Chapter Nine). Table 5–1 summarizes some procedures that require simple and informed consent.

Inadequate consent, also called "ignorant consent," is the opposite of informed consent. It may extend into simple consent, because it is not clear what type of information must be provided before consent can be assumed. When consent is not obtained, the legal consequence is usually battery; when consent is deficient or inadequate, the charge most often is negligence.

HISTORY OF CONSENT

Legal History

Simple consent has long been recognized as necessary for medical procedures. The case of *O'Brien v. Cunard Steam Ship Co.* (1891) found that a ship's passenger's action of getting in line to have an injection constituted implied

TABLE 5–1
EXAMPLES OF CONSENT REQUIREMENTS
FOR VARIOUS EXAMINATIONS

Simple Consent	*Informed Consent*
Routine radiography such as chest, extremities, and so on.	Contrast radiographic examinations such as barium enema, excretory urography, angiography.
Rationale: Considered noninvasive, low risk due to low dose*; few alternatives available (e.g., for fracture of an extremity, radiography is the accepted diagnostic tool). An exception would be radiography of a pregnant patient, which would require informed consent.	*Rationale:* Invasive, risks are increased (although in many cases still relatively low).
Abdominal ultrasound	Transvaginal ultrasound
Rationale: Noninvasive and low risk.	*Rationale:* Invasive procedure.
	All radiation therapy
	Rationale: Uses high doses of radiation, which has the possibility of side effects (including death, although side effects are typically benign). There are treatment alternatives, such as chemotherapy and surgery.
	All nuclear medicine
	Rationale: Invasive, injecting a radioisotope into body; public fear of terms "radioisotopes" and "nuclear" (associated with high doses of radiation), even though doses are low, may be a contributing factor.

*There are risks associated with low doses of radiation, although the chances of an effect are low and do not occur in the short term (e.g., cancers with long latent periods). Low doses of radiation as an invasive agent remains undiscussed, although imaging modalities such as ultrasound and magnetic resonance imaging are recommended at times due to the fact that they do not use ionizing radiation.

consent.[1] Since the passenger joined the line voluntarily, could see the act being performed, and was free to withdraw at any time, consent was given voluntarily.

The concept of informed consent can probably be traced back to the 1914 decision handed down in the *Schloendorff* case, in which Justice Cardozo stated, "Every human being of adult years and sound mind has a right to determine what shall be done with his own body; and the surgeon who performs an operation without his patient's consent commits an assault for which he is liable for charges."[2]

Informed consent as a doctrine can be traced to the 1957 case *Salgo v. Leland Stanford University Board of Trustees*.[3] In that case, the following was stated: "A physician violates his duty to his patient and subjects himself to liability if he withholds any facts which are necessary to form the basis of an intelligent consent by the patient to the proposed treatment." The central issues of informed consent come from the 1972 case *Canterbury v. Spence*.[4] The patient must be given information that indicates the risk, benefits, and alternatives of suggested treatments. Also, the outcomes that could result if a recommended treatment is not accepted must be provided.

A recent case, *Arato v. Avedon*, affirmed that the process of informed consent is to be seen as information-sharing, with the patient making the decision and the physician acting as a fiduciary to the patient. A fiduciary is one who handles the affairs of another. This relationship implies an element of trust, and if that trust is violated, the physician is liable.

In *Arato v. Avedon*, the California Supreme Court affirmed an appeals court decision that physicians were liable to disclose statistics concerning life expectancy to patients to allow them to take timely action to plan for death.[5] Without such information, the physician, rather than the patient, is making the treatment decision, and as Annas[6] notes, "this is precisely what the doctrine of informed consent is designed to prevent."

The Patient Self-Determination Act (PSDA) of 1990, which took effect in December 1991, mandates that health-care institutions receiving Medicare and Medicaid funding provide written information about patients' rights to participate in medical decision making and the formulation of advance directives.[7] Each state:

> "acting through a State agency, association, or other private nonprofit entity [must] develop a written description of the law of the State (whether statutory or as recognized by the courts of the State) concerning advance directives that would be distributed by providers or organizations under the requirements of [the Act]."[8]

The Tuskegee Experiment

In 1972, a news story broke detailing the exploitation of more than 400 African-American men who, suffering from syphilis, were left untreated but were followed up by medical professionals for 40 years. The study began in 1932, before antibiotics were available to combat the disease; however, when antibiotics became an accepted method of treatment in the 1940s, they were not offered to the subject group.[9] One official of the Centers for Disease Control (CDC) called the experiment "genocide," and analogies were drawn to Nazi medical experiments on Jewish prison camp internees.[10] The Tuskegee experiment was especially atrocious as it was long-term and nontherapeutic (no positive outcome could result from not treating the disease).

This is a classic case of not obtaining informed consent. The subjects in the study were not provided with information that would have probably led any reasonable person to seek antibiotic therapy. One cited legacy of the Tuskegee experiments is African-Americans' mistrust of the public health system, and more recently, of prevention programs for AIDS.[11]

Health professionals participating in the study have been seen as ethically liable. For example, nursing experts have found that nurses should have provided the patients with information about treatments available. Eunice Rivers, a public health nurse responsible for recruiting and retaining subjects, stated that during her training nurses were taught never to question doctors' orders.[12] This argument has not been accepted by the nursing community. Health-care professionals are ethically obligated to provide patients with treatment alternatives when these are in the patients' best interests.

DISCUSSION QUESTION
Use of information gained in studies such as the Tuskegee experiment and Nazi and Japanese medical experiments during World War II remain an unresolved ethical dilemma. Caplan notes that syphilis has proved to be a "stubborn and resilient" disease, and that the Tuskegee experiments have provided us with at least 13 articles and 4 books that help us in fighting this disease.[13] He asks whether, in retrospect, we should dismiss this information, or as he states, is "bad ethics bad science?" What is your opinion on this issue?

The Radiation Experiments

A number of radiation experiments were conducted in the 1940s through the 1960s without obtaining what today would be considered adequate informed consent. These experiments have special ethical relevance since they targeted groups that are considered vulnerable—women, children, the terminally ill, members of minority groups, and the indigent.[14] Consider the following:

- One reason why we know more about the radiation dose required to sterilize men as opposed to women is because of a study sponsored by the Atomic Energy Commission (AEC) in the 1960s. The study was conducted at Washington State Prison by researchers from the University of Washington. Sixty-four inmates were exposed to various doses of radiation (up to 600 rad or 6Gy) to the testicles. A similar study was conducted in Oregon. A consent form was signed in the studies (the inmates also received $200 and warnings about sterility and radiation burns), but inmates were *not* warned about the risk of testicular cancer.
- Researchers sponsored by the AEC and Quaker Oats fed radioactive iron and calcium to residents at the Fernald school for retarded boys, from 1946 to 1956, to see if cereal would block the absorption of the isotopes. Although doses were low, in some cases parents were only told that their children were singled out for a special program without mentioning radioactivity.

- Researchers at various sites in the 1940s injected 18 terminally ill men and women with plutonium to see where it would go in the body. Not until the 1990s did many family members even know that plutonium was used.[15] A direct analogy with the Tuskegee experiment can be drawn here because there is no therapeutic value to plutonium.
- A study at Vanderbilt University fed more than 800 pregnant women radioactive iron to establish nutritional guidelines during pregnancy.

Although adequate guidelines, such as the Nuremberg Code (Appendix A), were available even in the late 1940s, they were not followed. In the 1960s, a process for using institutional review boards (IRBs) was established to ensure that adequate measures are taken to secure informed consent in experimental studies. Outrage over the Tuskegee experiments led to the National Research Act of 1974, which then mandated IRB approval of all federally funded proposed research with human subjects.[16] However, there are a number of problems that still exist.[17] First, IRB members are usually colleagues of the individuals conducting the research, leading to potential conflicts of interest. In addition, because research dollars could be lost if studies are not approved, there is little incentive to not approve a study.

Also, IRBs only examine procedures and the forms (Appendix B). Consent is a communication process between a health-care professional and the patient (or researcher and subject). There is still concern today that physicians don't take time to adequately explain the ramifications of a study or indeed to communicate with their patients (Box 5–1).

Radiologic science professionals must understand that radiation used properly is a great tool; used improperly, it can cause harm to the patient. Radiation exposure is a risk versus benefit consideration—when used properly, radiation improves the health of the population. However, there are also small risks involved in radiation exposure. As the dose decreases, risks

---

Box 5–1. PHYSICIAN AND PATIENT COMMUNICATION

Much of the material in this chapter may seem to be overly critical of the physician and his or her communications with the patient. Is this justified? A 1982 study found that 96% of Americans wanted to be told if they had cancer, with 85% also claiming that they wanted a realistic estimate of how long they had to live if they were expected to live less than 1 year.[18] However, few physicians in that study would give patients full information regarding their condition; 13% stressed that they did not know how long a patient had to live and 28% said that it was generally less than 1 year. Studies conducted since that time have confirmed these results. Ten percent of physicians still do not tell their patients that they have cancer if they feel it would be detrimental to the patient's condition.

Johnson and associates[19] found that medical students had roughly the same problems as graduate physicians in securing consent, when such consent involved conflict. They recommend a number of interventions to help medical students learn how to involve patients in their own decision making.

decrease until at some point the risk might be zero. However, just as one must secure consent to inject a drug, one must secure consent to apply ionizing radiation to a human being.

One analogy for the medical imaging professional to consider is the pharmacist's situation. Pharmacists dispense prescriptions written by physicians, but they also consider themselves patient educators in helping the patient to understand the various actions and side effects of medications. Similarly, medical imaging professionals, who administer an agent (ionizing radiation) that has the potential for both benefit and harm, have certain responsibilities when acting as the physician's agent.

DISCUSSION QUESTION
The following comment was made by Rosalyn Yalow, a Nobel prize recipient for the use of radioisotopes in medicine:
"The large dose of radioactive iodine received by President Bush for the treatment of his overactive thyroid is not considered a problem. I, therefore, wonder why the radiation exposure in experiments a half century ago, which resulted in radiation exposure less than the president received . . . is a matter of current concern."[20]
Do you agree with the statement? What is the difference in President Bush's exposure and that of the patients in the experiments? Do you believe that there is a "safe" dose of radiation? Explain the rationale behind your answer.

DISCUSSION QUESTION
Suppose that you were asked to participate in a research study in your department that would expose patients to additional films to evaluate the use of a new piece of equipment. Based on the material you have just read, what types of questions might you ask to ensure that acceptable standards for consent were being followed?

SECURING CONSENT FOR IV CONTRAST PROCEDURES

Bush[21] notes that the use of informed consent for contrast media administration is not uniform throughout the medical imaging field. At one time, it was believed that it was best to allay patient fears about the procedure; it was accepted that patients would not want to know the risks of procedures using intravenous contrast.[22,23] This is no longer the case because of changing patient attitudes.

Another factor that must be considered is the use of nonionic contrast, a medium that provides fewer reactions but is much more expensive than conventional ionic agents.[24] In a limited resource environment, the ethical question arises of whether universal use of such an agent is justified. The financial resources required could perhaps be better used for other programs, such as child immunization. Bush notes that patients should be informed of the possibility of using the nonionic agents; he bases his opinion on what is known as a reasonable-patient standard, discussed below.

Standards vary among states in terms of the need to secure consent when using IV contrast. There are two basic standards: reasonable physician and reasonable patient. One state uses the standard of subjective patient.[25] The reasonable-physician standard used in most states will hold the physician responsible for "generally accepted" practice. That is, if most physicians in that state do *not* secure consent, the physician does not have to secure consent from the patient. The reasonable-patient standard holds the physician responsible for disclosing what a reasonable patient wants to know, rather than what a reasonable physician should disclose. Oklahoma uses a subjective-patient standard, which allows patients, at the time of trial, to say that they would have rejected the procedure based on nondisclosed risks. In both reasonable-patient and subjective-patient standards, written consent should be secured.

Box 5–2 contains a sample consent form for a contrast material injection developed by Bush. It is clear and readable and offers patients the information they should have to make an informed decision. These forms vary greatly among institutions. It must be stressed that consent should never be viewed simply as a form for patients to sign. Whenever patients have questions, they must be answered by the physician or the physician's agent.

> **DISCUSSION QUESTION**
> Secure copies of informed consent forms used in local clinical settings. Evaluate these forms. Ask medical imaging professionals at these sites what their role is in securing informed consent. Does this vary between facilities?

HOW IS CONSENT SECURED?

Two criteria must be satisfied for informed consent:

1. The individual giving consent must fully understand:
   - The nature of the procedure
   - The risks involved; including complications and side effects
   - Desired outcomes of the procedure
   - Possible alternatives

Box 5–2. SAMPLE CONSENT FORM FOR CONTRAST MATERIAL INJECTION

Your doctor has scheduled you for an x-ray examination that requires injection of a contrast agent in your bloodstream. As you know, an x ray is a picture of the organs and structures inside your body. The contrast agent (also termed contrast media, or contrast material, or "x-ray dye") shows up white on x-ray film or CT scan images and helps the radiologist interpret the x rays or CT scans.

The contrast media is given through a small needle placed into a vein, usually on the inside of your elbow or on the back of your hand or through a catheter if angiography is being performed. Normally, contrast media is considered quite safe; however, any injection carries slight risks of harm, including injury to a nerve, an artery, or a vein, infection, or reaction to the material being injected. Occasionally, a patient will have a mild reaction to the contrast agent and develop sneezing or hives. Uncommonly (one case in a thousand), a serious reaction to the contrast occurs. The physicians and staff of the x-ray department are trained to treat these reactions. Very rarely (1:40,000), death has occurred related to contrast administration; the risk of such a severe consequence is similar to that from the administration of penicillin.

Certain patients are at higher risk for experiencing a reaction to the contrast agent, and we are advising those patients to receive a different, more expensive contrast agent called "low osmolar" or "nonionic" contrast, which does appear to have a lower incidence of reactions; however, these newer agents are not absolutely free of reactions, even serious ones.

Patients who are at higher risk for adverse effects of contrast are:
1. People who have already had a moderate or severe "allergic-like" reaction to contrast material which required treatment
2. People with severe allergies or asthma
3. Patients with severe or incapacitating heart disease
4. Patients with multiple myeloma, sickle cell anemia, polycythemia, or pheochromocytoma
5. Patients with severe kidney disease, particularly that caused by diabetes

If you believe you are in one of the above categories, please notify the medical imaging professional or physician so that a nonionic or low-osmolar contrast agent can be used. Unfortunately, these agents are very expensive (an additional $90 to $130 per examination), and your insurance may not cover the additional cost.

If you are not in one of the high-risk groups, we recommend use of the standard or conventional ionic contrast agent for your x-ray study. These conventional agents have a long record of safety and effectiveness.

If you have any questions, please ask the attending medical imaging professional or radiologist to answer your questions.

I have read the above information and have had my questions answered.

(signed) _____

Name _____

Date _____

2. The individual giving consent has the legal capacity to do so if he or she is a(n):
   - Competent adult
   - Legal guardian or representative of an incompetent adult
   - Emancipated, married, or mature minor
   - Parent or legal guardian of a child
   - Individual obligated by court order

Health-care workers have a variety of legal and ethical responsibilities in securing consent. For example, physical therapists have developed an expanded role in consent over many other health professionals because of their ability to engage in independent practice.[26] Nurses have also continued to examine their role in consent, especially in the absence of a physician.[27] Inlander and Weiner[28] found that 83% of nurses were informing patients about alternatives to procedures when they felt that the physician had not done so.

Similarly, articles in medical imaging periodicals and journals have asked whether the medical imaging professional—as an agent to the physician—can secure informed consent, and they have examined circumstances that may hinder securing informed consent.[29,30] Radiologists have noted that their brief encounters with patients are inadequate for securing informed consent. Since the medical imaging professional spends more time with the patient and may be responsible for securing a patient history, this opens a potential role for the medical imaging professional beyond securing simple consent.[23] Some guidelines for the medical imaging professional are summarized in Box 5–3.

Box 5–3. GUIDELINES FOR MEDICAL IMAGING PROFESSIONALS IN SECURING CONSENT[29,30]

1. The procedure should always be explained in simple terms to the patient. The patient should agree to have the procedure performed. Silence is not agreement from a legal standpoint. Since one role of a medical imaging professional is to advocate for the patient, there should be a brief attempt to persuade the patient; however, coercion is unacceptable.
2. Resecure consent when taking over from another medical imaging professional. This is achieved by indicating who you are and that you intend to continue with the examination.
3. Procedures should be terminated whenever the patient expresses a desire to do so.
4. Consent should never be a ritual; it is a two-way process between patient and health professional. Questions that the medical imaging professional cannot answer must be referred to the radiologist or other physician.
5. Departments that allow medical imaging professionals to secure consent should have clear policies as well as in-service training to ensure consistency.
6. There are some examinations that do not lend themselves to having the medical imaging professional secure consent. These are examinations with a high risk and/or those which prompt patient questions that cannot be adequately answered by the technologist.

DISCUSSION QUESTION

Refer back to the pertinent code of ethics in Chapter Three. What is the principle in your professional code that might limit your role in securing patient consent?

DISCUSSION QUESTION

Consider the following aspects of consent that must be understood by the patient:

1. The nature of the procedure
2. The risks involved, including complications and side effects
3. Desired outcomes of the procedure
4. Possible alternatives

Research an examination that uses contrast, and role play with another student as the patient. What kinds of problems arose? How could you best address these? At what point did you feel it best to refer the patient to a physician?

CASE STUDY

THE PAUSCHER CASE[31]

Becky Pauscher delivered her first child on August 2, 1982, after entering Iowa Methodist Medical Center the previous day. Ms. Pauscher was scheduled to be released on August 6, but she developed a fever and pain in her right side. She was also discharging large amounts of blood in her urine. Her obstetrician consulted a urologist, who suspected a urinary tract infection and ordered an excretory urogram (EXU) for August 8.

Two shift nurses had informed Ms. Pauscher that she was going to have an EXU. One told her that she could have a mild reaction, for example, hives, or a severe reaction such as difficulty in breathing. The other nurse described only the possibility of a mild reaction, "just the warmth of the dye, that sort of thing." These discussions were charted only after the patient's death. No physician told either nurse to speak with Ms. Pauscher. No physician told the patient that severe reactions could include the possibility of death. Also, neither nurse asked Ms. Pauscher if she consented to the procedure.

The radiographer asked Ms. Pauscher before the procedure if she had any allergies. Supposedly, the nurse noted on a requisition slip that she had none. This slip could not be found. Later it was found that the chart contained evidence of allergies (bee stings) and that the patient had suffered from asthma as a child. The radiographer also neglected to ask the patient if she consented to the procedure but did tell her some of the minor complications that could occur. The radiologist present in the department did not see the patient.

After some of the contrast had been injected, the patient began to scratch her face. The radiographer stopped the procedure, looked for other "distress signs," and seeing none, continued with the injection. No hives were seen, but when the patient complained of severe chest pains, the radiographer again stopped the injection and summoned the radiologist. Ms. Pauscher died despite resuscitation attempts. The autopsy revealed that the patient died of anaphylactic shock.

The patient's husband sued the urologist and radiologist for failing to inform his wife that the contrast medium could cause a fatal reaction, contending that she could not give *informed* consent without that knowledge. He also charged the hospital with failing to establish procedures for informed consent.

The Court considered the risk of the contrast and whether this particular patient would have considered the nondisclosed information significant to affect her decision. The trial judge granted the physicians' motion for a directed verdict* because Mr. Pauscher had failed to provide expert testimony that the physicians had deviated from normal standards of care by not telling Ms. Pauscher about the remote risk of death associated with an EXU (about 1 in 100,000 to 1 in 150,000). The judge granted the hospital's motion for a directed verdict on the same grounds.

An appeals court affirmed the trial judge's ruling, but disagreed with his reasoning. These physicians *were* responsible for informing the patient of risks, but a jury could not have reasonably concluded that the "extremely remote" risk of death was significant to Ms. Pauscher or that it would have affected her decision to undergo the test. Similarly, since hospitals do not practice medicine, they are not required to inform patients of matters that pertain to the physician-patient relationship.

The appeals courts second ruling may no longer hold because of the decision in *Tobias v. Winkler* (4th District 1987, Illinois), in which it was established that hospitals may have a duty to require physicians to advise patients of risks associated with certain procedures, though they are not required to ascertain the validity of information or themselves inform the patient of the risk.[33] This case would require the hospital to have a consent procedure and provide consent forms.

Though from a legal standpoint, the physicians and hospital "won" this case, certainly no health professional acted wisely in the Pauscher case or communicated well with the patient. No one viewed consent as an opportunity to discuss the proposed procedure with the patient in detail, learn the patient's fears, and give the patient an opportunity to gain some confidence in the individual who was going to perform the procedure. From an ethical standpoint these professionals were clearly remiss.

---

*"When a trial judge decides either that the evidence and/or law is clearly in favor of one party or that the plaintiff has failed to establish a case and that it is pointless for the trial to proceed further, the judge may direct the jury to return a verdict for the appropriate party. The conclusion of the judge must be so clear and obvious that reasonable minds could not arrive at a different conclusion."[32]

> **DISCUSSION QUESTION**
> How could the Pauscher situation have been handled in a way that would have possibly prevented Ms. Pauscher's reaction and death? Analyze the case from the viewpoint of (1) communication, (2) ethics, and (3) law.

CONCLUSION

Consent exists on a continuum ranging from simple consent for a routine examination to informed consent for an invasive procedure. It requires appropriate communication with and education of the patient, a recognition of legal rights and obligations, and attention to the various ethical dilemmas that may arise. Medical imaging professionals have well-defined roles in simple consent. Along with other health professionals, they are also developing new roles in securing informed consent.

REFERENCES

1. O'Brien v. Cunard Steam Ship Co., 154 Mass 272, 28 NE 266 (1891).
2. Schloendorff v. Society of New York Hospitals, 211 NY 125, 126, 105, NE 92, 93 (1914). ˙
3. Salgo v. Leland Stanford Board of Trustees, 154 Cal Apl 2d 560, 317p 170, 1957.
4. Canterbury v. Spence, 464 F 2d 772, DC Cir (1972).
5. Arato v. Avedon, 13 Cal 4th 1325, 11 Cal Rptr 2d 169 (1992).
6. Annas, GJ: Informed consent, cancer, and truth in prognosis. New England Journal of Medicine 330:223, 1994.
7. Teno, JM, Sabatino, C, Parisier, L, et al: The impact of the patient self-determination act's requirement that states describe law concerning patients' rights. The Journal of Law, Medicine, and Ethics 21:102, 1993.
8. Patient self-determination act, in the Omnibus Budget Reconciliation Act of 1990, PL 101–508, sections 4206, 4751, enacted November 5, 1990.
9. Byman, B: Out from the shadow of Tuskegee: Fighting racism in medicine. Minnesota Medicine 74(8):15, 1991.
10. Jones, JH: Bad Blood: The Tuskegee Syphilis Experiment. New York, Free Press, 1981.
11. Thomas, SB, and Quinn, SC: The Tuskegee syphilis study, 1932 to 1972: Implications for HIV education and AIDS risk education in the Black community. American Journal of Public Health 81:1498–1505, 1991.
12. Vessey, JA, and Gennaro, S: The ghost of Tuskegee. Nursing Research 43:67,1994.

13. Caplan, AL: Twenty years after. The legacy of the Tuskegee syphilis study. When evil intrudes. Hastings Center Report 22(6):29–32, 1992.
14. Public protests spark "witch-hunt" fears over radiation experiments. Nature 367:303, 1994.
15. Elliott, M, Waller, D, Glick, D, et al: America's nuclear secrets. Newsweek, December 27, 1993, 14.
16. Faden, R, and Beauchamp, T: A History and Theory of Informed Consent. New York, Oxford, 1986.
17. Past radiation experiments may lead to new efforts for informed consent. Hospital Ethics, March/April 1994, 13–15.
18. President's Commission for the Study of Ethical Problems in Medicine and Biomedical and Behavioral Research: Making Health Care Decisions: The Ethical and Legal Implications of Informed Consent in the Patient-Practitioner Relationship. Vol 2. Washington, DC, Government Printing Office, 1982.
19. Johnson, SM, Jurtz, ME, Tomlinson, T, et al: Teaching the process of informed consent to medical students. Academic Medicine 67:598, 1992.
20. Doctors say tests on humans no threat. Birmingham News, February 9, 1994, 7D.
21. Bush, WH: Informed consent for contrast media. American Journal of Roentgenology 152:867, 1989.
22. Alfidi, RJ: Controversy, alternatives, and decisions in complying with the legal doctrine of informed consent. Radiology 114:231, 1975.
23. Spring, DB, Winfield, AC, Friedland, GW, et al: Written informed consent for IV contrast-enhanced radiography: Patients' attitudes and common limitations. American Journal of Roentgenology 151:1243, 1988.
24. Bettman, MA: Radiographic contrast agents—a perspective. New England Journal of Medicine 317:891, 1987.
25. Reuter, SR: An overview of informed consent for radiologists. American Journal of Roentgenology 148:219, 1987.
26. Coy, JA: Autonomy-based informed consent: Ethical implications for patient noncompliance. Physical Therapy, 1989, 826.
27. Davis, AJ: Clinical nurses' ethical decision-making in situations of informed consent. Advances in Nursing Science 11(3):63, 1989.
28. Inlander, CB, and Weiner, E: Take This Book to the Hospital With You. Allentown, Pa, People's Medical Society, 1993.
29. Dowd, SB: Issues in patient consent. Radiology Management 13(4):40, 1991.
30. Dowd, SB: Patient Consent. Albuquerque, NM, American Society of Radiologic Technologists, 1994.
31. Pauscher v. Iowa Methodist Medical Center, Jeff Watters and John Bardole, 408 NW 2d 355 Iowa (1987).
32. Pozgar, G: Legal Aspects of Health Care Administration, ed 5. Gaithersburg, Md, Aspen, 1993, p. 549.
33. Tobias v. Winkler, 156 Ill App 3d 886, 509 NE 2d 1050, 109 Ill Dec 211 4th District (1987).

APPENDIX A

Nuremberg Code

The great weight of the evidence before us is to the effect that certain types of medical experiments on human beings, when kept within reasonably well-defined bounds, conform to the ethics of the medical profession generally. The protagonists of the practice of human experimentation justify their views on the basis that such experiments yield results for the good of society that are unprocurable by other methods or means of study. All agree, however, that certain basic principles must be observed in order to satisfy moral, ethical, and legal concepts.

1. The voluntary consent of the human subject is absolutely essential. This means that the person involved should have legal capacity to give consent; should be so situated as to be able to exercise free power of choice, without the intervention of any element of force, fraud, deceit, duress, over-reaching, or other ulterior form of constraint or coercion; and should have sufficient knowledge and comprehension of the elements of the subject matter involved as to enable him to make an understanding and enlightened decision. This latter element requires that before the acceptance of an affirmative decision be made by the experimental subject, there should be made known to him the nature, duration, and purpose of the experiment; the method and means by which it is to be conducted; all inconveniences and hazards reasonably to be expected; and the effects upon his health or person that may possibly come from his participation in the experiment.

The duty and responsibility for ascertaining the quality of the consent rests upon each individual who initiates, directs, or engages in the experiment. It is a personal duty and responsibility which may not be delegated to another with impunity.

2. The experiment should be such as to yield fruitful results for the good of society, unprocurable by other methods or means of study, and not random and unnecessary in nature.

3. The experiment should be so designed and based on the results of animal experimentation and the knowledge of the natural history of the disease or other problem under study that the anticipated results will justify the performance of the experiment.

4. The experiment should be so conducted as to avoid all unnecessary physical and mental suffering and injury.

5. No experiment should be conducted where there is a prior reason to believe that death or disabling injury will occur; except, perhaps, in those experiments where the experimental physicians also serve as subjects.

6. The degree of risk to be taken should never exceed that determined by the humanitarian importance of the problem to be solved by the experiment.

7. Proper preparations should be made and adequate facilities provided to protect the experimental subject against even remote possibilities of injury, disability, or death.

8. The experiment should be conducted only by scientifically qualified persons. The highest degree of skill and care should be required through all stages of the experiment of those who conduct or engage in the experiment.

9. During the course of the experiment, the human subject should be at liberty to bring the experiment to an end if he has reached the physical or mental state where continuation of the experiment seems to him to be impossible.

10. During the course of the experiment, the scientist in charge must be prepared to terminate the experiment at any stage, if he has probable

cause to believe, in the exercise of a good faith, superior skill and careful judgment required of him, that a continuation of the experiment is likely to result in injury, disability, or death to the experimental subject.

APPENDIX B

Expedited Review: The IRB Application (University of Alabama at Birmingham)

(PLEASE TYPE)

Principal Investigator: ——————————————————————

Title of Project: ————————————————————————

——————————————————————————————————

Please indicate by checking the appropriate space below the category or categories into which you believe your project falls:

_____ (1) Collection of hair and nail clippings, in a non-disfiguring manner; deciduous teeth; and permanent teeth if patient care indicates a need for extraction.

_____ (2) Collection of excreta and external secretions including sweat, un-cannulated saliva, placenta removed at delivery, and amniotic fluid at the time of rupture of the membrane prior to or during labor.

_____ (3) Recording of data from subjects 18 years of age or older using noninvasive procedures routinely employed in clinical practice. This includes the use of physical sensors that are applied either to the surface of the body or at a distance and do not involve input of matter or significant amounts of energy into the subject or an invasion of the subject's privacy. It also includes such procedures as weighing, testing sensory acuity, electrocardiography, electroencephalography, thermography, detection of naturally occurring radioactivity, diagnostic echography, and electroretinography. It does not include exposure to electromagnetic radiation outside the visible range (for example x rays, microwaves).

_____ (4) Collection of blood samples by venipuncture, in amounts not exceeding 450 milliliters in an eight-week period and no more often than two times per week, from subjects 18 years of age or older and who are in good health and not pregnant.

_____ (5) Collection of both supra- and subgingival dental plaque and calculus, provided the procedure is not more invasive than routine prophylactic scaling of the teeth and the process is accomplished in accordance with accepted prophylactic techniques.

_____ (6) Voice recording made for research purposes such as investigations of speech defects or subjects responses to questioning.

_____ (7) Moderate exercise by healthy volunteers.

_____ (8) The study of existing data, documents, records, pathological specimens, or diagnostic specimens.

_____ (9) Research in individual or group behavior or characteristics of individuals, such as studies of perception, cognition, game theory, or test development, where the investigator does not manipulate subjects' behavior and the research will not involve stress to the subjects. Research involving sensitive matters such as sexual or political behavior *may* require full review. Expedited review *is not* appropriate if the subjects' responses, if known outside the research, could place them at risk of civil or criminal liability or damage their financial standing or employability.

_____(10) Research on drugs or devices for which an investigational new drug exemption or an investigational device exemption is *not* required. NOTE: The Board may request full review if in their opinion the subject will be at greater than minimal risk.

Attach a specimen or drug release form where applicable and a copy of any questionnaire to be used. Attach a copy of the Expedited Human Subjects Protocol located in this Guide.

SIGNATURE OF	DATE	DEPARTMENT	BUILDING
INVESTIGATOR			
		ROOM	PHONE

This space for IRB use only.

Reviewer's comments:

SIGNATURE OF REVIEWER   DATE

Expedited Review: The Human Subjects Protocol

(PLEASE TYPE)

Title of Project _____

_____

A. General Information

  1. Investigator

    a) Name of Principal Investigator _____

       Signature of Principal Investigator _____

       Date _____

       Department _____ Phone _____

       Building _____ Room _____

       Qualifications of Investigator _____

       _____

    b) List the name, rank, and major departmental appointment of other investigators participating in this project, if any.

       NONE _____

       OTHERS _____

       _____

    c) If medical supervision is necessary, give the name of the physician who will be responsible for supervision.

       _____ Phone _____

  2. Type of Proposal or Activity: ( ) New   ( ) Renewal

    Date of Last IRB Approval _____

    If this proposal is part of a grant, please indicate the following:

    Name of Grant: _____

    _____

    Principal Investigator of Grant: _____

  3. Source of Funds—State specific name of funding source.

Governmental Agency or Agencies _____

Foundation(s) _____

Corporation(s) _____

Individual(s) _____

None (   )

Internal (   ) UAB Departmental Funds

B. Number and Type of Subjects and Controls

1. Number of Subjects and Controls _____

_____

2. Type of Subjects and Controls _____

_____

3. Populations from which Derived _____

_____

4. Location of Study _____

5. None of the following _____, or including:

   Minor Under

   14 years of age   _____   Prisoners   _____

   Fetuses   _____   Mentally Retarded   _____

   Abortuses   _____   Mentally Disturbed   _____

   Pregnant Women   _____

   If any of the populations above are involved, attach a statement indicating the reasons for using these groups.

6. Will any of the subjects be from the Veteran's Administration Hospital?

   Yes _____   No _____

7. Other Institutions?

   Will any of the subjects be from other hospitals or institutions?

   Yes _____   No _____

   Name of Institution(s) _____

C. Duration of Study

   Probable duration of entire study _____

Total amount of time each subject will be involved _____

Duration of each phase in which subject will be involved _____

D. Abstract of the Research Plan

    1. Briefly describe the objectives and methodology of this project in lay language.

       Do not exceed the space provided.

       _____

       _____

       _____

       _____

       _____

       _____

       _____

       _____

       _____

       _____

       _____

    2. Risks and Precautions: List any possible risks—physical, psychological, and social.

       Describe any special precautions to be taken to avoid these risks.

       _____

       _____

       _____

       _____

_____

_____

_____

3. Confidentiality: Describe the procedures to be used to maintain confidentiality.

_____

_____

_____

_____

_____

_____

_____

_____

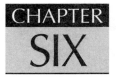

The Chemically Dependent Colleague

Rebecca W. Lam, MEd, ARRT(R)

Better living through chemistry and through technology may be a euphemism for less living, less awareness, less presence of mind and being. . . . We must respond to the diminishment of the self by helping to heal workers across the nation and around the world. Try spreading this message. There is a good chance that employers and employees will begin to listen, because the time has come for us all to change. It will cost us too much not to.—Angela Brown Miller, *Working Dazed*

Chemical dependence in health-care professionals is an established fact, yet medical imaging professionals have very little formal training about this disease. This chapter provides an overview of chemical dependence and its prevalence in the medical imaging professions. The influence of drugs on behavior and the reasons for chemical dependence are discussed. Ethical and legal issues are addressed; suggestions are given for actions to take if you suspect that a colleague or you, yourself, may be suffering from chemical dependence. A list of resources for getting help is also provided.

OBJECTIVES

At the end of this chapter, the reader will be able to:

- Differentiate impairment, alcoholism, and drug dependence
- Understand how chemical dependence has been viewed in the recent past and what is being done now to assist those in the workplace with this problem

- Describe reasons for chemical dependence and how drugs influence behavior
- Discuss key ethical and legal issues surrounding chemical dependence in the medical imaging professions
- Summarize procedural elements involved in recognizing and dealing with a chemically dependent colleague
- Identify alternatives for securing assistance if you suspect you are suffering from chemical dependence
- Given hypothetical scenarios, explore your values regarding chemically dependent colleagues and determine what your obligation is as a professional and co-worker
- List resources that will be helpful with chemical dependency issues

TERMINOLOGY

Alcoholism. Drug abuse. Addiction. Overdose. Medical imaging professionals have long been familiar not just with these terms, but also with the victims. Through their patients, medical imaging professionals have seen firsthand the effects of chemical substance abuse. It is logical to think that such experiences would make medical personnel refrain from abusing chemical substances, but that is not the case. Numerous studies over the years have confirmed the existence of chemical substance abuse by health-care professionals in medicine, nursing, dentistry, and pharmacy. In recent years, chemical substance abuse and dependence among medical imaging professionals have been documented.[1-3] The scope of the problem, coupled with increasing public attention and concern over safety, makes a full understanding of chemical dependence important for all medical imaging professionals.

Medical imaging professionals do not need to know all the pharmacological and behavioral aspects of chemical dependence to address the problem, but a well-rounded understanding of the terminology associated with this concept is essential. The term "impaired professional," which has been used to describe those with chemical substance problems, focuses on the person's inability to perform for a variety of reasons, not solely on those related to chemical substance abuse. Physician impairment was defined in 1972 by the American Medical Association's Council on Mental Health as "the inability to practice medicine with reasonable skill and safety to patients by reason of physical or mental illness, including alcoholism or drug dependence."[4]

The Merck Manual provides the following definition of alcoholism: "a chronic illness of undetermined etiology with an insidious onset, showing recognizable symptoms and signs proportionate to its severity."[5] It divides those with alcohol dependence into three categories: social drinkers, social alcoholics, and alcoholics. Social drinkers use alcohol as part of their socialization process, rarely become intoxicated, and do not tolerate drunkeness.

Social alcoholics are described as frequently intoxicated, but able to maintain some behavioral controls. Their excessive drinking does not significantly affect their marriages or interfere with their work. Alcoholics are those whose intoxication interferes with their ability to work and socialize. Their excessive drunkeness may lead to "marriage failure, being fired from a job, driving while intoxicated, medical treatment, physical injury, arrests, hospitalization."[5]

There is no single definition for drug dependence because of the different effects of various drugs. *The Merck Manual* does define "addiction," which encompasses drug dependence and involves an overwhelmingly compulsive use of a drug.[5] This implies the risk of harm and the need to stop the drug use whether the user recognizes the problem or not.[5] *Merck* describes three categories of drug abuse. Experimental or recreational users use drugs partially because they think it is culturally acceptable; they use relatively small doses, precluding any toxicity or dependence. Psychologically dependent users use drugs to find relief from, or insight into, their problems. Physically dependent users use drugs for a "high," and once they become dependent, continue to use them to prevent discomfort or withdrawal.

Regardless of drug choice, chemical dependence is characterized by loss of control and negative consequences associated with its use. Although many people feel chemical dependence is a moral defect or the lack of willpower to stop using drugs, chemical dependence is classified as a primary disease. The American Medical Association designated alcoholism as a disease in the 1950s, and today chemical dependence is also considered a primary disease that requires treatment.[6]

HISTORICAL REVIEW

Chemical substance abuse and dependence can be traced throughout our country's history, along with numerous attempts to control drug and alcohol use. The founding of Alcoholics Anonymous (AA) in 1935 by a physician and a stockbroker is considered a pivotal historical event because it paved the way for many of the self-help groups and treatment organizations that followed.[7] In the 1940s, occupational alcoholism programs (OAPs) were launched. They were the precursors to today's employee assistance programs (EAPs). It is thought that a meeting between Bill W. Wilson, co-founder of AA, and Maurice Dupont Lee, chairman of E. I. DuPont de Nemours, fueled the idea for an occupational alcohol assistance program.[8] Interestingly, E. I. DuPont was credited with the first multiplant OAP, and Eastman Kodak with the second, both in 1944.[9] By the 1970s, hundreds of corporations had started assistance programs, and the focus had shifted away from monitoring alcoholism symptoms and toward monitoring deteriorating work performance. By the 1980s, business groups had universally accepted the idea that chemical dependence resulted in employee increases in tardiness, absenteeism, accidents, job turnover, health insurance claims, and decreases in productivity and judgment. To counter these negative effects, thousands of major businesses and corporations initiated EAPs to assist employees with drug and alcohol treatment as well as other personal problems.

In the health-care workplace, employers lagged behind in recognizing the existence of chemical dependence. Professional organizations first brought the problem to light. In the 1970s and 1980s physicians and nurses, respectively, took the lead in actively addressing this problem in their own professions.[10,11] In 1982, pharmacists adopted formal policies and guidelines relating to professional impairment, particularly chemical dependence.[11] These professions overtly moved from a punitive posture to one of active support for an effective treatment and prevention process. They subsequently documented the use and prevalence of chemical substance abuse in their professions. Professional organizations then used this information to establish programs primarily through existing state organizations to assist chemically dependent colleagues.

Only recently have hospitals, the largest employers of health-care workers, begun to change their attitudes about chemical dependence. According to E. J. Holland, past chairman of a substance abuse task force for the American Hospital Association, hospitals were forced to change because chemical dependence was increasing.[12] Additional impetus resulted from increased awareness of hospital board members who, as businessmen themselves, were finding the need to address similar problems in their own workplaces. This led to the development of assistance programs that have now become a norm in health-care institutions.

CHEMICAL DEPENDENCE AMONG HEALTH-CARE WORKERS

Although the public has shown increasing concern about drug use in the general U.S. population, it has become even more apprehensive about those who provide public service, including health-care professionals. It has been speculated that health-care professionals may be different from the general population with respect to drug use because of multiple factors: (1) the effect the professional environment has on use; (2) the type or types of drugs used; (3) the probability of someone prone to chemical dependence choosing a "helping" profession; and (4) the influence of health education on drug use.[13] It has been conjectured that the health-care environment may make those who work in it more apt to use drugs because the high stress in this field is coupled with easy access to drugs, although relatively little documentation has been found to link stress directly with drug use or dependence. A recent study of resident physicians showed a higher correlation of drug use to strain, or reactions to the work environment, than to stressors, which are the stressful job conditions themselves.[14] This same study also revealed that benzodiazepines, (e.g., Valium), used predominantly for antianxiety or sleep-inducing purposes, were more strongly related to strain than other substances, intimating that self-treatment may be a concern among this group. Such pharmaceutical coping, or tendency to use some sort of drug to fix a problem that develops, potentially appears to be a greater issue among health-care professionals in general than stealing or diverting drugs, which may be more characteristic of select professions because of increased accessibility.

Prevalence and choice of drugs varies in the different health-care occupations, and even within specialties of a given profession. However, alcohol use and dependence have been repeatedly documented in the literature, indicating that alcohol is likely to be universally used and abused by all the professions. This is not surprising since alcohol is legal, and even drunkeness is moderately accepted by our culture. The literature also documents use of and dependence on other drug types, but data are conflicting even within a given specialty or profession, allowing no collective conclusions to be drawn.

It has also been theorized that people who choose a "helping" profession are more likely to have backgrounds characterized by dysfunctional families. In families that have been disrupted, children may assume a caretaker's role, which spills over into adulthood. When these people choose a profession, they have a tendency to pick a helping or service-related one, which includes the health-care occupations. Evidence to support this theory has not been absolute, but points in that direction.

Most educational programs in the health professions include pharmacology courses that focus on pharmacokinetics and pharmacodynamics. These courses may give students the impression that they have a good understanding of "drugs," and that this will prevent their use of drugs from developing into dependence. We are all familiar with the expression "a little knowledge can be dangerous," and this is certainly the case here. Recommendations have been made, especially in the last 5 years, that educational programs in the health professions focus on drug misuse, abuse, and dependence not only for patient counseling and referrals, but also for self-education.[15–19]

Is drug use among health-care professionals different from that in the general population? The U.S. population's drug use is known. It has been tracked since 1974 through the National Household Study on Drug Abuse (NHSDA), administered initially by the National Institute on Drug Abuse (NIDA) and currently by the Substance Abuse and Mental Health Services Administration (SAMHSA). Table 6–1 summarizes the NHSDA estimates of chemical substance use by the U.S. population in 1993.[20] All statistics, except for alcohol and tobacco, indicate nonmedical use only. Past estimates of alcoholism and drug abuse or dependence in the general U.S. population were 10% and 2%, respectively.[13] More accurate data from the National Institute on Alcohol Abuse and Alcoholism (NIAAA) in 1994 showed that

TABLE 6–1
INCIDENCE (IN %) OF CHEMICAL SUBSTANCE USE
IN U.S. POPULATION—1993[20]

Drug	Used in Lifetime	Used in Past Year	Used in Past 30 Days
Alcohol	83.6	66.5	49.6
Cigarettes	71.2	29.4	24.2
Smokeless tobacco	12.8	4.0	2.9
Any illicit drug	37.2	11.8	5.6
Marijuana	33.7	9.0	4.3
Cocaine	11.3	2.2	0.6
Any psychotherapeutics	11.1	3.8	1.3
Hallucinogens	8.7	1.2	0.2
Stimulants	6.0	1.1	0.3
Analgesics	5.8	2.2	0.7
Inhalants	5.3	1.0	0.4
Tranquilizers	4.6	1.2	0.3
PCP	4.1	0.2	NA
Sedatives	3.4	0.8	0.3
Crack	1.8	0.5	0.2
Heroin	1.1	0.1	NA
Anabolic steroids	0.4	0.1	NA
Needle use	1.4	0.3	NA

7.41% of the general population was either abusing or dependent upon alcohol.[21] This study did not acquire similar figures for other drug abuse or dependence, but other 1994 estimates showed that 5 million people (approximately 2% of the population) needed treatment for drug problems, and 41 million (approximately 16.5%) were dependent upon nicotine.[22]

Although research has indicated that chemical substance use among health-care professionals equals or exceeds societal patterns, this has not been proven. Most health-care studies have relied on self-report measures, producing data sets that are not as representative of their respective populations as the federal agency studies, which used personal interviews. Those surveyed, suspicious of the study's motives, may not have responded or been truthful. Others, because of memory problems associated with certain drug use, or because of simple lack of accurate recall, may not have responded accurately. Still others who were chemically dependent may have sincerely denied their state altogether, since denial is the hallmark of this disease. For these reasons, these studies have illustrated conservative estimates of use and dependence and produced some conflicting results, preventing their concensus. What *has* been accurately quantified is that most disciplinary cases in nursing and medicine that have come to the attention of the respective regulatory boards in the past have been related to chemical substance use or dependence.[13–23] Did these represent the majority of chemically dependent professionals in these groups? Not according to Sullivan,[13] who notes that, among recovering physician and nursing groups, few had been brought before their respective boards.

Prevalence of chemical substance abuse among radiologic science professionals has only recently been formally studied. In 1992, a broad health survey of radiographers included an assessment of technologists' use of cigarettes and alcohol.[24] With an overall response rate of 79%, 52.5% indicated having ever smoked 100 or more cigarettes, 46.7% were still smoking at the time of the study, 41.7% reported smoking one-half to one pack a day, and 28% stated that they smoked more than one pack a day. This same study showed that 82.1% of the radiographers drank alcohol, with 4.7% consuming more than 10 drinks a week.

In 1994, a study group (n = 249) comprising radiographers, diagnostic medical sonographers, radiation therapists, nuclear medicine technologists, and CT/MRI technologists employed by hospitals in a metropolitan area were surveyed using a slightly modified version of the NHSDA used by the federal government.[2] With a response rate of 55.8%, this self-report revealed that 83.5% had used at least one of the chemical substances surveyed in their lifetime, excluding childhood sips, puffs, and so on. It also confirmed that they used both legal and illegal substances and that the respondents' behavior was influenced by drug use.

In 1995, a random sample (n = 1913) of registered radiographers, sonographers, radiation therapists, and nuclear medicine technologists in Georgia were surveyed using the same survey tool as in the previous study.[3] The response rate was 35.3%, with 92.1% of the respondents self-reporting the use of chemical substances in their lifetime. Like the 1994 study, it showed that both legal and illegal substances were used, and that the respondents' behavior was influenced by drug use. Table 6–2 compares the prevalence of nonmedical drug use by radiologic science populations to national and regional populations using data from the three studies.

The top four drug types in the 1994 study were reported to be alcohol, tobacco, analgesics, and marijuana, in descending order of frequency. Nonmedical use during the respondents' lifetime of analgesics, stimulants, sedatives, and tranquilizers was markedly higher in the medical imaging population than in the general public. Use during the respondents' lifetime of cocaine, hallucinogens, and heroin was somewhat higher in the medical imaging population, and similar type use for alcohol, marijuana, and crack was somewhat lower in the medical imaging population. Cigarette and smokeless tobacco use was markedly lower in the medical imaging group than in the general population. However, of the substances that the study group had tried to cut down on, they reported having the least success with cigarette use.

The top four drug types in the 1995 study were alcohol, tobacco, marijuana, and cocaine, in descending order. With the exception of alcohol, overall percentage use of the other three drug types was lower in the 1995 study

TABLE 6–2
**INCIDENCE (IN %) OF NONMEDICAL CHEMICAL SUBSTANCE
USE IN LIFETIME OF U.S. AND REGIONAL POPULATIONS
COMPARED TO RADIOLOGIC SCIENCE (RS) POPULATIONS**[2,3,20]

Drug	1993 National	1993 Regional	1994 RS Study	1995 RS Study
Alcohol	83.6	80.3	76.3	80.8
Cigarettes	71.2	70.6	44.6	47.9
Smokeless tobacco	12.8	14.2	5.8	3.7
Marijuana	33.7	31.2	30.9	27.2
Cocaine	11.3	9.4	15.8	11.1
Hallucinogens	8.7	7.6	10.8	4.8
Stimulants	6.0	5.2	18.0	7.9
Analgesics	5.8	5.3	33.1	7.5
Inhalants	5.3	4.7	4.3	3.2
Tranquilizers	4.6	4.2	19.4	3.1
Sedatives	3.4	3.3	9.4	2.5
Crack	1.8	1.7	0.7	1.2
Heroin	1.1	0.8	1.4	0.9

than in the 1994 study. Nonmedical use of analgesics and stimulants was higher in this study group than in general and regional U.S. populations. The study population's cocaine use was lower than the general national average, but higher than the regional average. Use of all other chemical substances by this study group was lower than that in general and regional U.S. populations. Both the 1994 and 1995 radiologic science studies showed higher overall lifetime use among the study group of analgesics and stimulants as compared to societal patterns, and lower use of alcohol, tobacco, marijuana, inhalants, and crack. Results differed between the two studies for overall lifetime sedative, tranquilizer, hallucinogen, cocaine, and heroin use, and are therefore considered inconclusive.

FACTORS IN CHEMICAL DEPENDENCE

Chemical substances have been used throughout history to alter moods, perceptions, and brain functioning. It is also known that, while some people have used them without dramatic or long-term effects, others are markedly affected and become chemically dependent, exhibiting loss of control and the other negative consequences associated with drug use. Those who use chemical substances do not desire or expect to lose control or develop a chemical dependency. The chemically dependent person is most likely to start using drugs for "recreational" reasons, usually in a social setting. The initial experience may not be pleasant, and that will be enough to dissuade some from experimenting again. For others, the camaraderie that goes along with drug use is more important, and regardless of the quality of the experience, they use the drug again. Still others have a very pleasurable experience and enjoy the chemical effect, reinforcing additional drug use. With continued use, some find that it creates an illusion that cannot be produced any other way. Those people use drugs so they can temporarily exhibit personal qualities that they do not normally feel they have, such as attractiveness, importance, and self-confidence. People also use drugs as an escape from negative feelings such as distress, anxiety, depression, sadness, and boredom. Finally, some people take certain types of drugs that are supposed to have specific positive effects, such as increasing their creativity, expanding their consciousness, or improving their productivity.

Chemically dependent individuals may be affected by many factors: denial of dependence, the belief that stopping the drug use is not possible, and predisposing and contributing conditions. There are also individuals who choose not to quit.

Denial

Some individuals with drug dependencies sincerely do not believe they have lost control. This denial is classically found with chemical dependence. They do not see what may be obvious to others—that their drug use is affecting their personal relationships, their financial status, their work performance, and their personal well-being. Although they may acknowledge their drug use, they will not accept the idea that they have lost control and are chemically dependent. They typically feel they can stop using drugs at any time, and may really intend to quit. However, as time goes on, they develop a greater tolerance for the drug or drugs, which means that they must use larger and larger amounts to achieve the same effect. This classic path of denial sends them down the road to chemical dependence.

Belief that Stopping Is Impossible

Individuals with a drug dependence may fear the cessation of drug use and the effects of withdrawal. In reality, the side effects of withdrawal vary from person to person and substance to substance, and their impact can be exaggerated, depending on the person's psychological association to withdrawal.[25]

Recent research indicates that chemical changes occur in the brain as a result of drug use and may play a significant role in craving and dependency.[26] Positron emission tomography (PET) studies have shown that alcohol, cocaine, and nicotine reduce glucose metabolism in the brain, and that there is an inverse relationship between euphoria and metabolism: the lower the metabolic rate, the higher the euphoria. Other studies have shown that certain drugs, especially cocaine, deplete dopamine in the brain.[26] Because the dopamine system innervates several areas of the brain that control reinforcement, impulsivity, and self-control, abnormalities in it change the way the brain responds. In the case of certain drug use, it is thought that a dysfunctional dopamine system is responsible for loss of control and induction of compulsive drug consumption.

Another element in people who believe they cannot stop their drug use centers around faulty conceptions. For example, people may think that if they abstain from drug use, they will not be happy or they will be in control *only* if they use drugs. Thus, stopping may be perceived as a threat to their false sense of security. Also, some may think they do not have the staying power to stop using drugs permanently, so why try? Of course, this is a self-fulfilling prophesy in that they lack faith in themselves, are not firmly committed to stop, and become helpless when confronted with such a challenge.

Voluntarily Choosing Not to Quit

What about those who choose not to quit? As signs and symptoms of chemical dependence begin to appear, some may attribute them to something else (e.g., deteriorating work performance may be blamed on increased employer demands rather than on the effects of drugs). Others may recognize that their problems are caused by chemical dependence, but they place more importance on drug use than on other values. Sometimes this is based on a false ranking of values. As their problems worsen, people may waver in their stand in favor of drugs. Others, although a minority, maintain drug use as their top priority, in spite of being aware of associated problems.

Predisposition and Socioeconomic Conditions

Other factors also play an important role in a person's predisposition to chemical dependence. It is thought that those who come from families in which a member, typically a parent, suffered from substance abuse or addiction are more likely to suffer chemical dependence. Various studies, including several in nursing, have supported this theory.[27-29] The nursing studies also indicate that those people tend to choose a helping profession because of their caretaking role in earlier years. Also, though stress has not been validated as a direct corollary to chemical dependence, it is recognized as a contributing factor. Daily hassles of life may at some point become too much for a person's coping system and can serve as an encouragement to use drugs to make it through the day. The health-care professions are generally identified as stressful, and the strains associated with them have been shown to promote drug use.[14]

Chemical abuse and dependence have also been correlated with socioeconomic problems. Those who become disillusioned with improving their quality of life through traditional means are more apt to turn to drugs, especially if they have developed basic beliefs of helplessness or hopelessness.[30] At the other extreme are the affluent members of society who become chemically dependent because of basic beliefs of being ineffective or socially undesirable.[31] They typically begin using drugs to maintain their high social status or to accentuate feelings of power, invulnerability, and attractiveness. A common thread in both socioeconomic extremes is a vulnerability to peer pressure.[32] Socioeconomic influence is specifically noted as a factor of drug use in both nursing and medicine.[19,33-34]

Impulsivity is considered a predisposing factor to chemical dependency.[25] Some people develop a pattern of automatically yielding to impulses, without any prior reflection or conscious thought. The relationship of impulsivity to drug use and dependence is obvious. Less apparent is what causes impulsivity. PET research concerning chemical processes of the brain may lend valuable future insight to this characteristic. Regarding the health professions, it is not known if people who choose helping professions are more prone to impulsive behavior.

Last, evidence has been found to link a genetic predisposition with chemical dependence. People with a family history of substance abuse problems have been found to be more likely than those without that history to develop chemical dependence.[35] There is also a genetic component of vulnerability to alcoholism, as demonstrated by twin and adoption studies.[36] Animal studies have shown that the genes that control serotonin activity may influence alcohol preference.[37] Are people with a genetic predisposition to chemical dependence more likely to choose a helping profession than a nonhelping profession? As with impulsivity, no answer to that question has yet been formulated.

In summary, there are various theories and facts about the causes of chemical dependence. What is most important to keep in mind is that misuse of drugs will create problems, including dependence.

EFFECTS OF DRUG USE ON BEHAVIOR

Psychoactive substances affect behavior and performance, either directly through the central nervous system or indirectly through their interaction with other behavioral systems. The cerebral cortex, which is the highest level of impulse conduction of the central nervous system (i.e., it receives impulses from all parts of the body via the spinal cord or brainstem), is composed of functional areas associated with sensory, motor, and cognitive abilities, and no drug use affects only one of these abilities.[38]

The magnitude of drug effects on behavior is logically expected to be greater with chronic drug use than with occasional or moderate drug use. Since the latter is more prevalent among employed populations, is there reason for concern about the effects of moderate use on work performance? Numerous studies have shown that in moderate, occasional drinkers, "hangover" effects were observed after substantial alcohol consumption, even after blood alcohol levels (BAL) returned to zero. Therefore, even if alcohol use is restricted to personal, nonworking hours, work performance may still be affected. Moreover, studies have shown that the amount of alcohol in just one cocktail affects performance and social behaviors that are relevant to workplace performance, especially aggressiveness.[39] Moderate alcohol consumption has also been found to affect business decision making. "Wining and dining" is not advisable because even relatively low BAL compromises recall of information and promotes risky decision making.[40]

Unfortunately, even though there are documented effects of occasional drug use on work performance, obvious job impairment may not manifest itself for months or years, depending on the drug or drugs used. What are the effects of *chronic* drug use, more indicative of chemical dependence, on the workplace? First, remember that those who are chemically dependent have higher rates of tardiness, absenteeism, accidents, inefficiency, negligence, medical and workers' compensation claims, and theft. These are directly linked to the chemically dependent employee, with quantifiable costs. However, there are also indirect losses to the workplace that include poor decision making, adverse effects on coworkers' morale and performance, replacement and training costs, and a compromised community image. Given that up to 25% of the U.S. population is chemically dependent on at least one drug type, and that most chemically dependent people are employed, it is indisputable that businesses stand to lose millions of dollars annually because of chemically dependent employees. In light of a declining public trust of the U.S. health-care system over the past decade, it has become incumbent upon health-care institutions to take a highly active position on chemical dependence. This is due not only to the high cost of dependence, but also to the idea that the health-care system should take a leading role in health promotion and disease prevention.

Employee assistance programs (EAPs) are now the primary mechanism through which health-care institutions provide assistance to chemically dependent and other troubled employees. Central to a successful EAP are a solid substance abuse policy to which all employees are oriented and a complete understanding by supervisory and managerial personnel of the EAP's purpose and functions. Thus, it is imperative that supervisory personnel be taught to be sensitive primarily to specific signs of deteriorating work performance and, subsequently, to any accompanying symptoms that are indicative of chemical dependence. With this type of a focus, supervisory personnel are not put in the position of being responsible for diagnosing the reason or reasons for the employee's compromised performance, which is certainly out of their realm of expertise. Rather, they are to be attentive to their employees' job performance and refer them to the EAP for assistance when it becomes apparent that the employee's work is being affected by personal issues.

SIGNS AND SYMPTOMS OF CHEMICAL DEPENDENCE

What are the warning signals to which supervisors and coworkers should be alert? First, there are some background indicators for which those with hiring responsibilities should be watchful. These may be revealed during an interview and include a history of frequent job changes (at the same location or at various locations), prior medical history that involved pain control, and a family history of substance abuse or dependency.

Once an employee is on the job, a variety of behaviors may be exhibited. It is important to note here that *all* employees may exhibit some of these behaviors occasionally. However, a pattern of performance over a period of time should be noted. It is also significant to note that a chemically dependent individual will protect job performance at the expense of every other dimension of his or her life.[23] Indeed, the suggested order in which injury occurs is family, community, finances, spiritual and emotional health, physical health, and *finally* job performance; therefore, observation of the following behaviors and their documentation is paramount in developing a globally accurate image.

Absenteeism is one of the most common behaviors. This includes tardiness, leaving work early, and frequent absences while at work. The latter may include unusually long breaks or lunches, frequent trips to the restroom, or places remote to their immediate work area, such as the operating room (OR) or emergency room (ER). Excessive sick leave, use of sick leave immediately after personal days off, repeated leaves of absence, unauthorized absences, and elaborate or improbable reasons for tardiness or absence are also to be noted.

Regarding technical job elements, supervisory personnel should look for inconsistent performance, poor decision making, unjustified mistakes, increased accidents, difficulty meeting schedules, request for night shift, and unreliability. For a given section's type of work, supervisory personnel should look for job shrinkage not only in terms of decreased productivity, but also in terms of decreasing complexity of cases or tasks performed. Interactions with coworkers may change and include aloofness, isolation from colleagues, eating alone, overall morale change, avoidance of superiors, increased need to borrow money, and complaints from coworkers. Personal behavior changes include moodiness, increased temper or aggressiveness, cockiness, jitters, nervousness, irritability, difficulty with concentration, forgetfulness, confusion in recalling specific information, tiredness, lethargy, slowed reaction time, daydreaming, and complaints about work, family or marriage.

Physical signs and symptoms include shakiness or hand tremors, slurred speech, watery eyes, constricted or dilated pupils, vacant staring, red eyes, runny nose, weight loss or gain, GI disturbances, headaches, poor muscle coordination, carelessness about personal hygiene and appearance, characteristic breath odors, tracks, and use of long-sleeved clothing in hot temperatures.

What if the person experiencing drug use problems is the supervisor or manager? Certainly, the indicators above apply, but there are other signs that may appear and are dependent on the level and type of management position involved.[41] At lower management levels, the supervisor may become less strict with supervisory responsibilities, let safety standards decline, give conflicting instructions, use employee time and skill ineffectively, and submit incomplete reports or data. At higher management levels, declining job performance is more subtle and may include poor or impaired decision making, mismanaged budgets, lack of coordination with scheduling, and failure to deliver proper service.

ETHICAL SCENARIO

You have been working in a diagnostic imaging department of a medium-sized hospital for several years. Over the past several months, you have noticed that one of your coworkers has developed the following work behaviors: decreased productivity, increased absenteeism, diminished physical appearance, runny nose, headaches, weight loss, and frequent absences while at work (i.e., going to the restroom more often than usual). You also caught two patient identification errors he made last month and several computer entry mistakes in the last several days. You are beginning to suspect that this person may have a "drug problem." What do you do?

INTERVENTION

When a medical imaging professional is put in a position of deciding whether to intervene in some way, his or her interpretation of what action to take is founded in large part on his or her own personal code of ethics. There are basically two major classes of ethical theories on which ethical codes are based: deontology and utilitarianism. Each individual's ethical code stems from these theories, but it is also based on a lifetime of experiences, as discussed in Chapter Two. Each person's ethical code provides him or her not with a set of rules or laws that must be followed in all circumstances, but with a guide that will generally hold true in most cases. On that basis, a person develops a set of morals, which are customs or actions, and accompanying rationales, that are believed to be right for a given situation. This is why an action that is taken by one person may not be considered ethical or moral by another, and underscores why ethical issues are so difficult.

A prime example is the scenario above, to which multiple basic ethical principles apply. Nonmaleficence, which means to inflict no harm, pertains because of the potential for patient harm from the technologist's mistakes. The principle of beneficence is relevant because of the question of whether the medical imaging professional's behavior is contributing to the good health and welfare of patients. Of course, the autonomy of the coworker in question or the person's right to decide his or her own course of life (another basic ethical tenet) may appear to be in direct opposition to the issues of nonmaleficence and beneficence. Other ethical dilemmas confront the medical imaging professional in this scenario: Veracity, which means telling the truth, applies indirectly here in the decision as to whether the supervisor should be told about the mistakes. There might be other mistakes that were not caught, raising another question about nonmaleficence. Asking the opinions of the other staff to get a better "feel" of the situation before saying anything to a supervisor might possibly create a confidentiality issue.

Usually, most people are elastic enough in their ethical standards to make judgments based on the merits of a given situation, such as the one above. In addition to personal ethical standards, the medical imaging sciences have ethical codes of conduct that may serve as guides in making decisions about professional conduct (see Chap. Three). Also, medical imaging professionals should be familiar with the American Hospital Association's "Patients' Bill of Rights," which expounds on what the patient has a right to expect regarding ethical practice in a hospital. Thus, the preceding scenario could be viewed as an issue of patients' rights versus the employee's rights. On one hand is the major concern of safety and well-being of patients under this technologist's care; on the other hand is a major concern for the employee's rights.

Across multiple professions there is the tendency of a colleague, given the preceding scenario, to say nothing and to "cover up." Why? Historically, this "conspiracy of silence" has boiled down to (1) not wanting to violate the autonomy of the medical imaging professional by unjustifiably labeling him or her, and (2) desiring to prevent a colleague from being disciplined. Add to that the fear of suffering either personal reprisals or legal action for violating the coworker's civil rights, and the result is inaction. However, the greatest problem of all may be ignorance about chemical dependence. This possibility has been raised by Sullivan,[42] who states that professionals surveyed about their awareness of others with chemical dependency recognize few such cases. They were correctly identified by only a relatively small group who either had been chemically dependent themselves or had worked in some area related to this disease. The inference is that if more professionals received formal education about chemical dependence, it would increase their ability to recognize a chemically dependent colleague.

Parallel to this is the issue of workplace policies. A lack of formal guidelines for dealing with chemically dependent employees persists.[43]

When forced to deal with a problem of chemical dependency, management has resorted to punitive measures, including termination, and commonly for peripherally documented reasons, as the following sadly details:

> Employers often attribute the termination to other causes rather than confront the real issue. Obvious though it may be, alcohol or other drug use may never be mentioned. One nurse reports she was found unconscious on the restroom floor with a needle in her thigh and she was fired for "being regularly late returning from lunch."[44]

If clearer, more articulate guidelines and policies were developed at the workplace for dealing with chemically dependent employees, it might sufficiently raise the comfort level of professionals to spur them to take appropriate action.

Not to be overlooked is the ethical responsibility of the person suffering from chemical dependence. Recognizing chemical dependence as a primary disease does not absolve him or her from any responsibility. Just as a person who is diagnosed as having had a myocardial infarction has a responsibility to accept the illness, modify his or her lifestyle, and follow a certain therapeutic regimen to improve his or her health and well-being, so too does the chemically dependent colleague. If the person is unwilling to take on that responsibility, then he or she cannot expect to divert disciplinary measures.

DRUG TESTING

This chapter would not be complete without mentioning drug testing. Substantial ethical debate exists about the accuracy and usefulness of laboratory testing for drug use. Urinalysis is the most common laboratory test used in the workplace to screen for drugs and will be the focus of this discussion. Urinalysis is used because it detects metabolites of drugs in the urine. When drugs enter the body, they are carried via the bloodstream to the liver, where they may be metabolized. Any unchanged drugs and their metabolites reenter the bloodstream and are filtered by the kidneys. The length of time a drug may remain in the body depends on the drug type, but it ranges from less than an hour to up to several months. Therefore, any unchanged drugs and metabolites that are in the body at the time a urine sample is collected is detected and identified by urinalysis.

Different methods can be used to run a urinalysis drug screen, including radioimmunoassay (RIA) and enzyme immunoassay (EIA); thin layer chromatography (TLC), used for initial screenings; and gas chromatography (GC) and mass spectroscopy (MS), used for comfirmatory testing. Generally, the more sensitive and accurate the methods (i.e., GC and MS), the more expensive, complex, and time-consuming they are. Accuracy depends on the collection and handling or "chain of custody" procedures of the specimen. This brings up a major ethical issue of drug testing—accuracy of results.

It is possible for the person being screened to deliberately sabotage the specimen to create false negative results. It is also possible to produce inaccurate results from the specimen being mishandled (e.g., if it is not stored at the correct temperature) or from using poorly trained personnel or laboratories that are not appropriately certified to perform forensic urine drug testing (FUDT). A laboratory that is certified by the College of American Pathologists (CAP) is not automatically certified to do FUDT. The laboratory should have a separate CAP-FUDT or NIDA certification. This requirement is not commonly known.

Another source of inaccuracy is drugs being legitimately taken by the person being screened. Both over-the-counter and prescription drugs can produce false positive results for certain drugs, so it is imperative that attention be paid to this when an initial drug screen comes back positive. Thus, it is possible to produce both false-positive and false-negative results if the screening process is not of the highest quality and painstakingly followed.

Another major ethical issue surrounding workplace drug testing is its usefulness. While drug screening determines the *presence* of certain drugs of abuse, it is not normally done in such a way as to indicate *amount*. Additionally, there is no correlation with job performance. In other words, some argue that even if a drug screen produces positive results, it does not demonstrate unacceptable job performance or chemical dependence. Certainly this is true when the drug test is being used as a preemployment screen. It may, of course, also be performed in a rarer "for cause" situation. In this case, a drug test is triggered when there is reasonable suspicion of employee drug use, abuse, or dependence because of certain on-the-job behaviors, incidents, or accidents.

Other ethical issues of drug testing include confidentiality of test results and use of specimens for detection of other conditions. The issue of confidentiality of the drug test results themselves is obvious—test results should be limited to only those staff that absolutely need to know. However, urine specimens could be used to detect not only presence of drugs, but also other confidential information, such as pregnancy status or other unrelated diseases or conditions. This not only raises ethical issues about confidentiality and consent, but also has legal implications, and it is important to address this in drug-testing policies. The bottom line of drug testing is that, if it is used, there should be a clear policy that supports the philosophy of the employer and instills confidence in the employees regarding its purpose, need, and confidentiality. Remember also that patients have a right to know about the quality and safety of the health-care services they receive. How many of us would suggest that patients interview every health-care professional with whom they come into contact, not only about the procedural quality and safety or risk, but also about the drug use of the employee or employees performing the service or procedure? Certainly, this appears ridiculous, but what is the alternative? Given this viewpoint, drug testing may be considered a reasonable option, as the following true story under-scores:

> A woman who worked in an addictions career went into labor and at an appropriate time, went on to the hospital. While her husband was down-stairs filling out paperwork, the L & D staff suddenly began preparing her for an emergency C-section. Her physician was not there, and alarmed, the woman began asking questions about the necessity of a C-section. The staff indicated the baby's heartbeat was dropping dangerously fast, and they needed to do a C-section. The woman then asked, "How many, if any of you, have used alcohol or any other drug in the last 48 hours? If you have, when, which drug, and how much of it?" All but one of the staff appeared shocked, and the remaining employee laughed awkwardly. No one answered the woman, but the C-section was not performed. Her healthy, normal baby was born by regular vaginal delivery.[45]

LEGAL ISSUES

When the public recognizes that generally held ethical principles and guide-lines are not followed, they typically call for more formal means of regulation. Hence, legal mandates are created and handed down. Such was the case when the Federal government responded to growing public concern in the 1980s by taking the lead in passing legislation related to drug use. One of the major pieces of legislation was the Drug-Free Workplace (DFWP) Act of 1988. Those employers who are awarded property or service contracts of at least $25,000 or more by a federal agency, individuals who enter into any other contract for any amount with a federal agency, and all recipients of federal grants of any amount are required under this legislation to:

- Publish a statement notifying employees that the manufacture, posses-sion, distribution, sale, or use of drugs is forbidden at work and that violations will result in disciplinary action; promptly inform the proper federal agency whenever an employee is convicted of a drug-related offense; and impose punitive measures upon employees who are convicted of drug-related offenses in the workplace (including options such as mandatory drug treatment or rehabilitation, suspen-sion without pay, or job termination)
- Provide educational programs that include general information on the dangers of drug abuse and specific information on the hazards of drug abuse in the workplace and on the availability of drug counseling services and drug treatment or rehabilitation programs
- Make a good-faith effort to maintain a drug-free workplace by imple-menting these requirements[46]

This act globally seeks to keep drugs and their influence away from the workplace. How that is specifically accomplished is up to the employer's particular DFWP policy. Probability of litigation is greatly influenced by the quality of the policy and the employees' perception of it. However, when a confrontation takes place, the best, most positively held policy will not prevent an employee from taking a defensive attitude, especially in light of potentially serious disciplinary action. Also, legal issues tend to be brought up more commonly in the public sector rather than in the private sector because more restrictions or statutes apply to the public domain. Some of the legal issues that may emerge when dealing with chemical dependence in medical imaging departments involve drug testing, search and seizure, and discrimination.

The employer's ability to prevent legal ramifications with drug testing is directly proportional to the design of the testing program and the specificity of testing policies. Drug testing programs may include preemployment, "for cause," automatic, or random screening designs. Those in both the public and private sector have charged that preemployment drug screening violates certain constitutional amendments related to privacy, self-incrimination, and due process.[47] These amendments do not bar drug testing, but do require guidelines that assure a reasonable intent (i.e., a safe worksite), fair process, and security of employee rights.

For-cause testing is used when there is reason to suspect that a particular employee exhibits signs or symptoms of chemical substance abuse or dependence. From a legal sense, it is recommended that supervisory personnel be trained to identify multiple types of signs—behavioral, observable, and physiological—to maximize support information.[47] Automatic testing is triggered by a given situation or incident. This type of testing is common in the transportation industry in that drug testing of appropriate personnel is automatically performed when some transportation service accident occurs. It can be found in health-care settings, but is more prevalent when there are discrepancies in drug counts or missing controlled substances, and is not a common practice in medical imaging settings.

The last category, random or periodic testing, has drawn the most fire. Most legal cases in the public sector have held random screening to be unconstitutional, and it remains an unclear area in the private sector.[47] This is based on the argument that there is no evidence or reasonable suspicion of employee impairment on which to justify testing. To minimize negative employee perception, some programs incorporate a modification of random testing in which employees are provided with a notice of intent to test. In this case, the employee would be informed of a time period during which testing may occur, referred to as a "window for testing" (e.g., October 1 through October 15). The employee can test negative if he or she abstains for an appropriate amount of time prior to, and during, that period.

Search and seizure is another legal risk area. Technically, drug testing is considered a form of search and seizure, but it can be legally performed under reasonable and fair policies. Other types of search and seizure may also be performed, but again these must be within the confines of a written policy that has been communicated to employees before such activity occurs and that is consistent with federal, state, and common law and reasonable business practice doctrine. Legal battles tend to center on an invasion of privacy issue. Employee claims of violation of constitutional or common law rights have been denied when care has been taken to notify employees of the policy at some previous time and, in cases of random searches, that the searches could include employees' vehicles parked on the employer's property and packages that employees carry on and off the employer's property.[47] Conversely, in the instance in which the employer has justifiable reasons to suspect an employee possesses or is under the influence of drugs at the workplace, but did not preannounce a search policy, the employer may conduct a search only of unconcealed items or areas where there is no privacy expectation.

The preceding discussion deals with property of the employee. Property that is provided by the employer, such as lockers, desks, and vehicles is a separate issue. Settlements for both the employer and the employee in cases involving searches of employer's property make it difficult to draw an absolute conclusion. However, case law leans toward the employer *if* there is an established policy indicating that the employer reserves the right to inspect lockers, desks, and other employer-owned property without consent. The rationale for this is that the employer has given the employee prior notice not to expect those areas to be considered private.

Another issue that has embroiled employers in legal battles is discrimination of job applicants who have histories of chemical dependence. In hiring considerations, employers are prohibited from discriminating against those who have recovered from chemical dependence as well as those who are currently undergoing supervised treatment. This protection is specifically cited in the Americans with Disabilities Act (ADA) of 1990.[48] Job prospects who are found to suffer from substance abuse or dependency at the time of application and who are not actively participating in some form of legitimate rehabilitation may not be considered.

In summary, whether the employer is required by law, as are DFWP participants, to have a substance abuse policy or whether it is by the employer's choice, the key is a well-written document that balances employee responsibilities and employee rights. It is common to find that legitimate legal issues surface because of ambiguous or unaddressed content or violation of other legal statutes. Authors of such substance abuse policies should be intimately familiar with civil rights and antidiscrimination legislation, tort law, labor law, and state statutes.

CONFRONTATION AND CARE IN THE MEDICAL IMAGING ENVIRONMENT

It is natural for a coworker or supervisor in the medical imaging field to express concern and to inquire as to what is wrong when a medical professional exhibits signs of distress. Typically, a professional in this situation offers an explanation and an apology for "being out of sorts." A chemically dependent employee may react in the manner just described, but is more likely to respond by denying the existence of a problem, blaming someone else, or shunning any form of help or concern. What is important to remember is that, with the chemically dependent coworker, this scenario will take place again and again.

The supervisor should, of course, review and adhere to all applicable policies and procedures at his or her institution for intervention with the chemically dependent employee. The following is a general protocol of actions and their sequence.

Procedures for Intervention

First, the supervisor should document as objectively and specifically as possible what the worsening job behaviors are. Depending on the supervisor's knowledge of, and experience with, department and institutional policies, he or she may consult the human resources department or the EAP for advice on how to best accomplish this. Next, the supervisor should speak with the employee. The supervisor should give thought to choosing a time and place when the medical imaging professional will be the most receptive. During this meeting, the supervisor should explain why it is taking place, including a statement of concern for the employee and his or her performance. The supervisor should then discuss the specific negative behaviors and the need to modify them. The supervisor should identify as specifically as possible what is expected of the employee and what consequences, if any, will occur if the medical imaging professional continues to exhibit unacceptable performance.

After this meeting, the supervisor should monitor the employee's behavior for an appropriate time period. The supervisor should then meet with the employee again to discuss whether the employee's performance has been appropriately modified. If this is the case, the supervisor should encourage the employee to continue this positive behavior. If the medical imaging professional has not improved acceptably, the supervisor should issue a warning that if he or she cannot reach a certain performance level within a given period of time, the employee may face the possibility of a discharge. The supervisor should offer an alternative course of behavior by encouraging the medical imaging professional to seek out the services of the EAP. The employee certainly does not *have* to do so, but must understand that if he or she continues to exhibit unacceptable performance, then disciplinary action will follow, with the distinct possibility that continued unsatisfactory progress will result in job termination.

If the employee accepts the referral to the EAP, then the supervisor should provide reasonable emotional support and any other practical assistance, making sure the employee understands that participating in the EAP will not exclude him or her from disciplinary measures if the employee's performance does not improve. If the medical imaging professional shows acceptable performance improvement, then the supervisor should continue to provide positive feedback. If the employee does not show acceptable performance improvement even with EAP support, the supervisor should counsel him or her that disciplinary action will follow, as discussed in the second interview. If the employee's performance does not improve after disciplinary action is taken, then the supervisor should proceed with termination. While this should be a last resort, it is essential to follow through with the procedure, or its integrity will be totally undermined. Of extreme importance is that accurate and objective documentation be maintained throughout the process. If the medical imaging professional is terminated, he may likely appeal the action, in which case the value of a written record that accurately reflects details cannot be overestimated.

Policy for Maintaining Recovery

If the employee successfully recovers from chemical dependence and his or her job performance returns to an acceptable level, it is logical to think this is the end of this process. However, with chemical dependence, sustained care is essential to maintain true recovery. After completing whatever primary treatment is necessary, the recovered medical imaging professional needs to continue with some form of treatment that might include periodic counseling, attendance at support group meetings, or "after hours" outpatient care. Again, the supervisor should follow the employer's policies and procedures, and should ensure that the medical imaging professional understands what is expected of him or her. For example, the policy may specify that a written agreement exist between the employee and the institution outlining the terms for continued employment and the consequences for violation of those terms. Thereby, both the institution and the employee are protected. The institution is assured that the employee is maintaining recovery, and the employee is assured that there is appropriate documentation precluding any suspicions of relapse and the need for extensive monitoring. The key to any policy is that an accurate assessment of the situation be made and reasonable support and opportunities for assistance be provided, allowing the institution to meet its obligation to the medical imaging professional, its staff, its patients, and the public.

CONCLUSION

The heart of the problem in dealing with any chemically dependent employee is the reluctance to get involved. However, chemical substance abuse and dependence, like other problems, are here to stay and will not go away unless something is done. Action is needed at professional, institutional, and individual levels.

First, chemical dependence needs to be accepted as a problem that deserves attention in the medical imaging profession. If perceptions are that, although *some* medical imaging professionals may suffer from this disorder, chemical dependence is not a significant problem in our profession, we are fooling ourselves. Although medical imaging professionals differ somewhat from the general population in use of specific drug types, drug usage parallels that of the U.S. population enough to develop estimates of chemical dependence in our profession. Statistically, that means that just under 19,000 formally credentialed medical imaging professionals may suffer from alcoholism, approximately 5100 may suffer from addiction to drugs other than alcohol, and some 42,100 may suffer from nicotine addiction. This does not take into account all the uncredentialed workers in the field. Thus, the word "some" may be more closely interpreted to be over 66,000 medical imaging professionals.

Barriers of ignorance need to be removed by developing educational offerings for both formal credentialing programs and employee continuing education programs about chemical dependence, including how to recognize its signs and symptoms. Specific guidelines are needed on how to deal with medical imaging professionals when their job performance deteriorates because of chemical dependence. Moreover, it should be emphasized that these guidelines should also apply to those in management. Research has repeatedly shown that professionals emulate one another, and if those in higher positions exhibit good values and morals, they are likely to see their staff and students imitating them.

Chemical dependence should continue to be studied by the profession, and both professional groups and employers should collaborate to discover the best methods for assisting medical imaging professionals who suffer from it. Much can be learned from other professional groups and businesses that have already blazed a trail for us to follow in designing an appropriate system to provide assistance to our ranks. Of course, future efforts would be incomplete without paying significant attention to prevention measures.

Finally, medical imaging professionals must change their attitude toward chemically dependent colleagues and show compassionate care to coworkers who need help.

The attitude that one person cannot make a dent in this problem grossly underestimates the difference an individual can make. Medical imaging professionals do not often know a patient's outcome, but that does not mean that their part in that person's care is any less significant. Likewise, medical imaging professionals may not appreciate the impact that they can have on those with whom they come into contact. A small gesture, like expressing concern to a chemically dependent coworker who appears resistant to any form of help, may make the coworker receptive to someone who comes along later with another offer of assistance. An individual can make a difference, as the following story shows:

> A visitor was walking along the beach when he noticed a man in the distance. As he got closer, he noticed that the man kept leaning down, picking something up, and throwing it in the ocean. As he continued walking, he realized the man was picking up starfish that had washed up on shore. As he approached the man, he asked him what he was doing. The man replied that it was low tide, and if the starfish that had washed up to shore weren't thrown back, they would die from lack of oxygen. The visitor, seeing the hundreds of starfish lying on the beach, indicated that the man couldn't possibly throw all of them back. "Can't you see that you can't possibly make a difference?" the visitor asked the man. The man smiled, picked up another starfish, and as he threw it back into the water, replied, "Made a difference to that one!"[49]

DISCUSSION QUESTIONS

1. A medical imaging professional, whom coworkers and the supervisor suspect of having an alcohol problem, appears at work with an alcohol smell on his breath, compromised gait, and slightly slurred speech. The supervisor pulls him aside, specifically identifies the signs he has outwardly observed, reminds the employee that, according to the substance abuse policy, this is grounds for drug testing, and requests that the employee undergo a blood test. The employee refuses to cooperate with his request. Is this insubordination, or would the testing be a violation of the professional's rights?

2. A medical imaging professional is given a copy of the institution's policies and procedures upon being hired. One year later, the employee begins showing signs and symptoms of a chemical dependency problem, including chronic tardiness, frequent absences from the work area, and excessive sick leave. The supervisor warns the employee about this behavior, but his behavior does not improve. The supervisor then counsels the medical imaging professional again and suggests that he avail himself of the institution's EAP services. The employee refuses, indicating that he has no problems that are affecting his work. After another week of similar behavior, the supervisor suspends the employee for 3 days without pay and warns him that continued behavior would result in termination. The employee states that the action was unduly severe. The supervisor states that the action was consistent with the institution's policies and procedures. The employee files a grievance, citing that although he was given a copy of the policies and procedures when he was hired, he had not reviewed them specifically since that time, and that

the supervisor was negligent not to have mentioned them in previous interviews. Who is right?

3. A medical imaging professional is charged with driving under the influence (DUI) and possession of marijuana while off duty one weekend. The local paper, which regularly prints all the DUI and drug-related violations once a week, identified the professional and the charges against him. Several days later, a patient he was imaging recognized his name from the drug violation list in the paper. The patient immediately halted the exam and asked for the supervisor. Upon meeting with the supervisor, the patient demanded that the medical imaging professional not be allowed to work there because of his drug-related charges and the negative impact it had on her ability to trust his work performance. What should the supervisor do?

4. A medical imaging professional who works for a mobile imaging company is given a company-owned vehicle to drive as part of his employment contract. The company begins receiving complaints from several of their clients that this professional is drinking on the job, and is also suspected of snorting cocaine while working. One day after work, a representative for the company goes to his house, where the company car is parked and requests to search the vehicle. The medical imaging professional refuses the request. Is this an ethical issue, a legal issue, or both? Who is right? Can an employee refuse to cooperate without risking being charged with insubordination or another similar policy violation?

5. A radiation therapist is approached by coworkers, who all express concern that she is showing signs of chronic alcoholism, including significant weight loss, "alcohol breath" early in the morning, chronic tardiness, frequent requests to leave early from work, and lowered productivity. The therapist flatly denies any possibility, but the coworkers consult the supervisor. The coworkers know that, shortly after that, the supervisor met with the therapist, but nothing appeared to happen. After the coworkers make repeated requests of the supervisor to deal with the therapist, with no overt action being taken, the coworkers each begin documenting particular events related to the therapist's work performance and behavior. Three months later, the therapist is found passed out at her console at work by a coworker. A blood alcohol test indicates almost toxic levels, and the therapist was terminated. She immediately sues the employer for not providing assistance with her drinking problem. All the therapist's coworkers are subpoenaed. Does the therapist have a legitimate case? What would you do if you were one of the cowork-

ers who had specific written documentation of the therapist's behaviors and had been told you were definitely going to be put on the stand?

6. You are a medical imaging professional whose employer does periodic random drug testing. You recently had a drug test at work. You were notified by your supervisor that the test came back positive and that discharge proceedings were being initiated. You have never used drugs, including alcohol and tobacco, in your life. What do you do?

7. A medical imaging professional, returning from a week's vacation, is requested to undergo a periodic random drug screen the day he got back. His urinalysis tests positive for marijuana. The employee states that he had smoked some "weed" while he was off, but is not impaired, and can function well in his position. If you were the supervisor, how would you handle this situation? Does the employer have a right to impose punitive measures? If you were the employee, what would you do if disciplinary action was taken?

8. Just after lunch, a medical sonographer performs a preliminary scan on a patient scheduled for an amniocentesis. When the physician comes in to begin the procedure, the sonographer notices that the physician's hands are shaking, his speech is slightly slurred, and there is a faint alcohol odor on his breath. He appears to be having difficulty with the needle puncture. If you were the sonographer, what would you do?

REFERENCES

1. Readers write. RS Wavelength 2(6):4,6, 1991.
2. Lam, R, Jense, J, and Etersque, S: Chemical Substance Use Among Radiologic Science Personnel: A Pilot Study. Journal of Nuclear Medicine Technology 24:59–64, 1996.
3. Lam, R, Jense, J, Reyes, L, et al: Prevalence of Substance Use Among Radiologic Science Personnel. Chemical substance use among RTs in Georgia. Radiologic Technology 67:501–512, 1996.
4. American Medical Association Council on Mental Health: The sick physician: Impairment by psychiatric disorders, including alcoholism and drug dependence. JAMA 233:684–687, 1973.
5. The Merck Manual, ed 15. Rahway, NJ, Merck Sharp & Dohme Research Laboratories, 1987, pp 1477, 1479.
6. Talbott, GD, Gallegos, K, Wilson, P, et al: The Medical Association of Georgia's impaired physicians program. JAMA 257(21):2927–2930, 1987.
7. Scanlon, W: Alcoholism and Drug Abuse in the Workplace—Employee Assistance Programs. New York, Praegar, 1986, p 14.
8. Ibid, p 21.
9. Target: Alcohol Abuse in the Hard-to-Reach Workforce. Rockville, MD, National Institute on Alcohol Abuse and Alcoholism, 1982, p 3.
10. Haack, M, and Hughes, T (eds): Addiction in the Nursing Profession. New York, Springer, 1989, pp x,xi.

11. Bissell, L, Haberman, P, and Williams, R: Pharmacists recovering from alcohol and other addictions: An interview study. American Pharmacy NS29(6):19–30, 1989.
12. Poteet, M: Wrongs vs. rights. RS Wavelength 2(5):1,12, 1991.
13. Sullivan, E: Impaired health care professionals. In Bennett, E, Woolf, D (eds): Substance Abuse, ed 2. Albany, Delmar, 1991, pp 293–304.
14. Jex, S, Hughes, P, Storr, C, et al: Relations among stressors, strains, and substance use among resident physicians. International Journal of the Addictions 27(8):979–994, 1992.
15. Sullivan, E, Bissell, L, and Williams, E: Chemical Dependency in Nursing—The Deadly Diversion. Menlo Park, CA, Addison-Wesley, 1988, p 20.
16. Aach, R, Girard, D, Humphrey, H, et al: Alcohol and other substance abuse impairment among physicians in residency training. Annals of Internal Medicine 116:245–254, 1992.
17. McNamara, R, and Margulies, J: Chemical dependency in emergency medicine residency programs: Perspective of the program directors. Ann Emerg Med 23(5):1072–1076, 1994.
18. Sheffield, J: The special needs of women pharmacists in recovery. American Pharmacy NS32(7):45–47, 1992.
19. Hughes, P, Brandenburg, N, Baldwin, D, et al: Prevalence of substance use among US physicians. JAMA 267(17):2333–2339, 1992.
20. Substance Abuse and Mental Health Services Administration, U.S. Department of Health and Human Services. National Household Survey on Drug Abuse: Population Estimates 1993. Rockville, MD, U.S. Department of Health and Human Services, pp 17, 23, 29, 35, 41, 47, 53, 59, 65, 71, 77, 83, 89, 95, 101–104, 1994.
21. Grant, B: Prevalence of DSM-IV alcohol abuse and dependence. Alcohol Health and Research World 18(3):243–248, 1994.
22. Lewis, D: The Need for Substance Abuse Treatment. Brown University, 1994.
23. Talbott, G, and Wright, C: Chemical dependency in health care professionals. Occupational Medicine: State of the Art Reviews 2(3):581–591, 1987.
24. Boice, J, Mandel, J, Doody, M, et al: A health survey of radiologic technologists. Cancer 69(2):586–598, 1992.
25. Beck, A, Wright, F, Newman, C, et al: Cognitive Model of Addiction in Cognitive Therapy of Substance Abuse. New York, The Guilford Press, pp 22–41, 1993.
26. D'Agincourt, L: Nuclear medicine aids clinical war on drugs. Diagnostic Imaging 15(6):87–90, 108, 1993.
27. Black, C: It Will Never Happen to Me. Denver, MAC Printing and Publishing, 1981.
28. Bissell, L, and Haberman, P: Alcoholism in the Professions. New York, Oxford University Press, 1984.
29. Sullivan, E: Comparison of chemically dependent and non-dependent nurses on familial, personal, and professional characteristics. Journal of Studies on Alcohol 48(6), 1987.
30. Beck, op cit, p 197.
31. Beck, op cit, p 198.
32. Beck, op cit, p 199.
33. Cronin-Stubbs, D, and Schaffner, J: Professional impairment: Strategies for managing the troubled nurse. Nursing Administration Quarterly 9:44–54, 1985.
34. Green, P: The chemically dependent nurse. Nursing Clinics of North America 24(1):81–94, 1989.
35. Beglieter, H, Porjesz, B, Bihari, B, et al: Event-related potentials in boys at risk for alcoholism. Science 211:1064–1066, 1984.
36. National Institute on Alcohol Abuse and Alcoholism. Eighth Special Report to the U.S. Congress on Alcohol and Health. Bethesda, Md, National Institutes of Health, pp 62–65, 1993.
37. Murphy, J, McBride, W, Lumeng, L, et al: Regional brain levels of monoamines in alcohol-preferring and -nonpreferring lines of rats. Pharmacology, Biochemistry, and Behavior 16(1):145–149, 1982.
38. Heishman, S, and Henningfield, J: Application of human laboratory data for the assessment of performance in workplace settings: Practical and theoretical considerations. In Drugs in the Workplace: Research and Evaluation Data, Volume II. Rockville, MD, National Institute on Drug Abuse, pp 167–174, 1991.
39. Kelly, T, Foltin, R, and Fischman, M: Effects of alcohol on human behavior: implications for the workplace. In Drugs in the Workplace: Research and Evaluation Data, Volume II. Rockville, MD, National Institute on Drug Abuse, pp 129–142, 1991.

40. Jobs, S: Impact of moderate alcohol consumption on business decision-making. In Drugs in the Workplace: Research and Evaluation Data, Volume II. Rockville, MD, National Institute on Drug Abuse, pp 147–161, 1991.
41. DeFeo, D: Alcohol/Drug Abuse: It's High Time You Knew the Facts. Meeting Planners International—Professional Education Conference, Anaheim, CA, December 7, 1993.
42. Sullivan, E, Bissell, L, and Williams, E, op cit., pp 15,19.
43. Haack, M, and Hughes, T, op cit, p 26.
44. Sullivan, E, Bissell, L, and Williams, E, op cit, p 24.
45. Miller, A: Drug testing: A test of will and right. In Working Dazed. New York, Plenum, 1991, p 96.
46. US Congress, 41, USC Sec 701 et seq, Drug Free Workplace Act of 1988.
47. Colosi, M: Substance abuse: Management responses. In Handbook of Health Care Human Resources Management, ed 2. Rockville, MD, Aspen, 1990, pp 519–534.
48. Texas Young Lawyers Association: The Americans with Disabilities Act—An Overview. 1990, pp 4–5.
49. Canfield, J, and Hansen, M: One at a time. In Chicken Soup for the Soul. Deerfield Beach, FL, Health Communications, 1993, p 22.

APPENDIX

Self-Assessment

What if you suspect you are suffering from chemical abuse or dependence? The first step in solving any problem is to recognize its existence. Several quick self-assessment tools can be used: two of these are the Michigan Alcoholism Screening Test (MAST),[1] which has short and long versions, and the CAGE questionnaire[2] used to assess alcoholism, which poses these four questions:

1. Have you ever tried to cut down on your drinking?
2. Have you ever been annoyed by criticism made by others about your drinking?
3. Have you ever felt guilty about your drinking?
4. Have you ever needed an "eye-opener" to get going the morning after a drinking bout?

These tools are not meant to function as definitive diagnostics but as general guides. If these measures indicate that your suspicions may be correct, you need professional assistance. Do not delay in obtaining help just because everything currently appears to be "okay." Remember that many heart attack victims also classically deny the seriousness of their symptoms, wait too long to get help, and subsequently find themselves in a fight for their lives. If your workplace has an EAP, it will be in your best interest to make an appointment with someone there who can counsel you appropriately. EAPs are designed to provide privacy, and they are frequently geographically distanced from the workplace, so that it is not common knowledge as to who avails themselves of their services. EAP services are also normally provided at no cost to the employee, unless it is found that long-term therapy or treatment is needed, in which case you may be referred to a more appropriate group or agency. If your workplace does not have an EAP or you do not feel comfortable using it, other sources of help exist and are listed below. In choosing a resource, it is advised that you pick one that deals specifically with chemically dependent individuals, and preferably one that is experienced in dealing with health-care professionals. General mental health groups may not have the best success with recovery from this disease.

Sources of Help

Alcoholics Anonymous (AA)
(212) 686-1100

Al-Anon Family Group Head-quarters
(212) 302-7240

Cocaine Anonymous
(213) 559-5833

Drug Abuse Information and Treatment Referral Line
1-800-662-HELP

Drug Free Workplace Helpline
1-800-843-4971

Families Anonymous
(818) 989-7841

Marijuana Anonymous
(213) 964-2370

Men for Sobriety, Inc.
Women for Sobriety, Inc.
(215) 536-8026
(separate organizations administered through one office)

Narcotics Anonymous
(818) 780-3951

National Council on Alcohol
(212) 206-6770

National Clearinghouse for Alcohol and Drug Information
1-800-729-6686

National Institute on Alcohol Abuse and Alcoholism
(301) 443-3860

National Institute on Drug Abuse
(301) 443-6245

For addresses and phone numbers of the listed organizations in your local area, please consult the yellow pages or call the number listed.

REFERENCES

1. Selzer, M: The Michigan Alcoholism Screening Test (MAST): The quest for a new diagnostic instrument. Am J Psychiatry 3:176–181, 1971.
2. Ewing, J: Detecting alcoholism: The CAGE questionnaire. JAMA 252 (14):1905–1906, 1984.

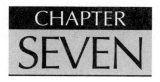

Special Populations
Steven B. Dowd, EdD, ARRT(R)

This chapter discusses the following issues of interest to medical imaging professionals: the legal and ethical aspects of child abuse and elder abuse, the obligation to report HIV status and to work with HIV-positive patients, and the rights of dying patients.

OBJECTIVES
At the end of this chapter, the reader will be able to:
- List ethical dilemmas that arise in the treatment of children
- Describe child abuse and the medical imaging professional's role in reporting child abuse
- Discuss the importance of maintaining autonomy in the elderly
- Describe elder abuse and the ethical dilemmas that result from the treatment of elder abuse victims
- Discuss ethical dilemmas surrounding the practitioner with HIV
- Discuss the medical imaging professional's ethical obligation to treat the HIV-positive patient
- Discuss death and dying, including active and passive euthanasia

CHILDREN

Two basic interrelated issues are present in the ethical treatment of children: (1) the child's ability to make informed choices and (2) the parent or guardian's "ownership" of a child. Verzemnieks and Nash[1] note that although the developmental level of the child may be more important, society has traditionally used age as the determinant for ability to make informed decisions. Thus one might be a child at age 17 years and 364 days but not at age 18.

Similarly, for many years parents and guardians were seen as the owners of children, and therefore able to make all their decisions. This attitude no longer holds, and now even children have some rights in making decisions. A further complication is the fact that many times an adult other than the parent or guardian, a grandmother or a teenage brother perhaps, might bring a child to the hospital. Such individuals may have no legal right to make treatment decisions for the child.[2]

DISCUSSION QUESTION

An ethical dilemma surrounds the rights of parents with specific religious beliefs to decide against medical intervention. A child arrives in the emergency room (ER) after a bicycle accident, and a subdural hematoma is suspected. You are the technologist assigned to perform computerized tomography of the head on the child. Suppose the child's mother, who had not previously been available, arrived and demanded that you cease scanning her child because she did not believe in hospital treatment and felt that "God should decide the child's fate." Although the decision whether to continue would not be made at your level (you would refer her to a physician), it is important that you clarify your own feelings about these situations in order not to become disillusioned with your job. How do you feel about these situations? Can a parent decide for a child? Do parents have the right to demand that children follow their religious beliefs (a "slippery slope" argument)? (See Box 7–1.)

Child Abuse

Radiography is an important tool in diagnosing child abuse. It is likely that you will encounter cases of child abuse, and you may be called on to report your findings. This depends on a variety of factors. You need to have a clear concept of what constitutes child abuse legally because this determines whether "mere suspicions" can be reported. For example, Arizona law requires that a report be made if injuries are not explainable based on available medical history, or if there are any other grounds to believe a child has been denied or deprived of necessary medical treatment or surgical care.[3]

There are three broad categories of reportable child abuse:

Box 7–1. THE "SLIPPERY SLOPE"

One well-known argument in ethics is the "slippery slope." It is based on the analogy of moving down a slippery slope, where a misstep may cause us to lose control until we are rapidly falling to the bottom. Similarly, any action that seems logical or without danger can end up supporting actions that are unacceptable. The slippery slope carries arguments to their extremes. For example, if we believe in active euthanasia, do we then kill anyone who we no longer find "useful?" What about the physically challenged? Anyone over age 70? Individuals we find to be "ugly?" If we support abortion, do we support parents who choose not to have a child simply because of its sex, which is done in some countries?

The slippery slope argument makes us aware of the possible consequences of a belief. It challenges our values by making us think about extensions of an argument that we may not have previously considered.

- Physical abuse—harm or threatened harm suffered by a child through nonaccidental injury as a result of acts or omissions of persons responsible for the care of the child.
- Sexual abuse—the commission of any sexual offense (usually described in the criminal code) with or to a child as a result of the act or omissions of the person caring for the child.
- Neglect—harm that occurs to a child through failure of the parent or caretaker to provide adequate food, clothing, shelter, medical care, or other provisions necessary for the child's health and welfare.[4]

Mandatory and Permissive Reporting

A "blanket" approach to mandatory reporting requires all persons to report.[5] For example, the New Jersey statute requires that "any person having reasonable cause to believe that a child has been subjected to child abuse or acts of child abuse shall report the same immediately."[6] In this state if the individual does not file, he or she can be held liable under a "disorderly persons offense" if there is "reasonable cause to believe that an act of child abuse has been committed." The Alabama code is similar, but slightly more restrictive, requiring reporting on the part of "any person called upon to render aid or medical assistance to a child."[7]

Many states (e.g., Colorado) are fairly general in the types of health-care personnel required to report. After physicians and nurses, "hospital personnel engaged in the admission, care, or treatment of patients," are listed as mandated reporters.[8] The Virginia code states that "any person licensed to practice medicine *or any of the healing arts* [author's emphasis] . . . who has reason to suspect that a child is an abused or neglected child shall report the matter immediately."[9] As radiographers are *not* currently licensed in the state of Virginia, they might not be considered mandatory reporters.

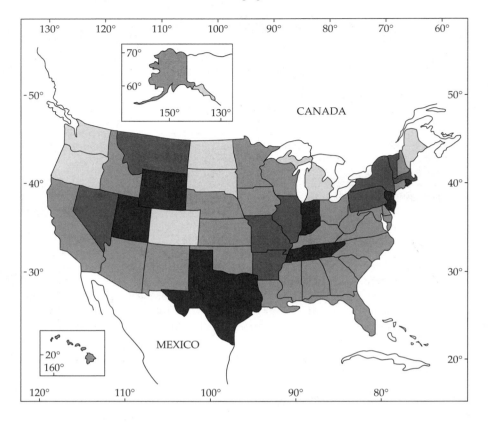

Key:

■ Anyone must report

▨ All medical professionals/personnel must report

▨ All staff members of health facilities must report

□ Legislation does not potentially include RTs

FIGURE 7–1.   State-by-state child abuse reporting mandates. In all states and the District of Columbia, all physicians, dentists, and nurses must report suspected child abuse.

West Virginia and Maryland have similar statutes and *are* licensure states.[10,11] Here radiographers are subsumed and can be required to report.

Most states require reporting on the part of various professionals in the course of their normal duties (Fig. 7–1). Some states, such as Oregon, however, require that child abuse observed in "any situation" be reported.[12] This increases the potential liability but blurs the clarity of each situation; for example, is a medical professional required to report an obviously malnourished infant seen in a department store?

Those who *may* report child abuse are called permissive or permissible reporters. For example, the District of Columbia code states that "in addition to those who are required to report, any other person may make a report."[13] Wisconsin statutes state that "any other person . . . having reason to suspect that a child has been abused or neglected, or reason to believe that a child has been threatened with an injury and that abuse will occur, may make such a report."[14]

Most states allow both mandatory and permissible reporting. It is important to know whether a professional group is covered under a mandatory statute because failure to report may result in criminal charges. In states where medical imaging professionals are considered mandatory reporters, they may also lose their license if they do not report. Failure to report under a permissible statute is not a crime. Permissible statutes are enacted to allow a broader range of reporters while still maintaining a group of mandatory reporters.

Immunity and Liability. Legal immunity is designed to protect reporters of suspected child abuse from prosecution. Because a civil suit for slander or libel may result from reporting, states have granted immunity to reporters to encourage frank and prompt reporting.

Absolute immunity is designed to protect individuals regardless of intent. In such cases there is a presumption of good faith. A New Jersey case held a physician immune from prosecution in a civil suit; it did not matter whether he acted out of malice or good intent.[15] Even in states without absolute immunity, successful suits against reporters are almost unheard of.

Approximately half of the states grant conditional immunity. In such cases good faith (that is, absence of malice or reporting for an ulterior motive) is assumed.

Reporting Procedures. Reporting varies according to two factors: hospital or institutional policy and state law. In New York State, for example, suspected abuse or neglect must be first reported by phone to the New York State Child Abuse and Maltreatment Register. A registry number that must be included in a follow-up report is provided. Blatant physical abuse and sexual abuse are considered criminal acts, reportable to police. A written report must be made to the State of New York Department of Social Services within 48 hours of the initial phone call.[16]

The following information is most important in reporting child abuse:

- Child's name and address
- Name and address of parent or caretaker
- Age of child and present whereabouts
- Details of the nature and extent of presenting injuries
- Evidence of previous injuries from scars or healing bruises
- Name, age, and condition of other children in the home

- Parents' or caretakers' description of injury
- If known, person responsible for injury, or name(s) of person or persons caring for child at the time of injury
- Statement summarizing reasons for suspicion of abuse

Most health-care institutions have clear, written reporting guidelines. An arrangement in which individual staff members can report their findings to a central committee is common. This allows each professional on the health-care team to contribute relevant information according to his or her involvement in the case and professional standing. Some states consider notification to a central committee fulfillment of the reporter's obligations. The reporter is not responsible if the committee does not make the report. In other states, the reporter may still be held liable if the report is not filed.

> **DISCUSSION QUESTION**
> Secure a copy of the child abuse law in your own state. What type of reporters are medical imaging professionals? Does the state grant conditional or absolute immunity for reporters?

CASE STUDY

SUSPECTED CHILD ABUSE

Sally Jones is a radiographer in a large, urban medical center. After performing a radiograph on a child with a fracture, the clinical signs, patient history, patient communications, and the radiograph lead her to suspect abuse. However, she is then told by one of the ER nurses that the child is the son of one of the most respected surgeons on staff, an individual who brings millions of dollars in business to the hospital each year.

Multiple healed fractures are present in addition to the new fracture. This may indicate a history of abuse. Sally wonders why this has not been previously reported. Possible reasons might include:

- Health professionals did not recognize their social and ethical responsibilities to report abuse. For example, some radiographers believe that their job is to take diagnostic radiographs and that they have no other responsibility to the patient. Health professionals are not always fully cognizant of their responsibilities on a social and ethical level.
- The father's position of power clouded the reasoning of health professionals previously working with the child. It would be

difficult to believe that a respected physician could be guilty of child abuse.
- The father was able to provide acceptable reasons for his son's injuries. We tend to trust, and usually with good reason, individuals in positions of authority and power. The father is probably able, based on his education, to give reasonable explanations for the injuries.

Sally is cautioned by the ER nurse, a friend of hers, to "leave well enough alone," and not report the abuse. Sally feels that if she does not make the report, she will not be fulfilling her role as an advocate to the patient, and she doubts whether she will be able to live with herself. She goes ahead with the report even though it may compromise her job.

OLDER PEOPLE

There are a number of moral and ethical issues related to the care of elderly persons. Most of these center around autonomy. Aging is a universal and irreversible process; all humans who live long enough experience a decline in their physical and mental abilities. For most individuals, these changes are not severe enough to bring about the need to be institutionalized. In fact, most elderly people are healthy enough to carry on the activities of daily living, perhaps needing just a little help. Simply because one takes longer to perform tasks does not mean that one is unable to do them; similarly, the normal forgetfulness that occurs with aging does not mean that one is "senile."

Most older people are able to make their own decisions. The need to put those decisions in the hands of others is an ethical dilemma: Has the person lost the ability to make logical decisions? Who should then decide? According to Watkins,[17] caregivers dealing with impaired elderly persons must perform a delicate balancing act between the rights of the individual and the risk older persons may pose to themselves and others. Niemira,[18] a primary care physician, believes that ethicists have ignored many of the true issues involved in the care of frail, incompetent elderly people, preferring to focus on popular topics such as active euthanasia. Health-care workers are trapped between being overly paternalistic and attempting to reforge patient autonomy (another example of the "slippery slope"). Physicians, for example, are unsure of what to do for patients in a compromised state who are neither curable nor dying.

Radiographers, according to the ASRT Code of Ethics, are expected to be, first and foremost, patient advocates. This is an outgrowth of the ethical principle of beneficence—to do good. Other imaging professionals (e.g., nuclear medicine technologists and ultrasonographers) are governed by similar codes, which are discussed in Chapter 3.

DISCUSSION QUESTION

Suppose an older patient comes to your department for a barium enema. The patient is having the examination against her wishes; she has been declared "incompetent." However, on speaking with her, you believe that she is able to, and should be allowed to, make decisions on her own. How do you proceed?

DISCUSSION QUESTION

Another issue related to the autonomy of elderly persons is the use of patient restraints. On the nursing unit, restraints are sometimes used by staff so that patients "can't hurt themselves." However, from an ethical and legal standpoint, restraints should only be used when all alternatives have been exhausted. Similarly, imaging professionals who, out of convenience, restrain patients who are able to cooperate, face legal charges and are in fact acting unethically. Discuss the proper use of restraints as well as alternatives to restraints to ensure that you will use them properly.

Elder Abuse

Recently, elder abuse has become more common. This could be attributed to increased life expectancy and more people having to care for their elders. It is also possible that we have simply become more aware of it and more willing to talk about it. There are five types of elder abuse:

1. Physical abuse
2. Financial abuse
3. Psychological abuse
4. Sexual abuse
5. Self-abuse and/or neglect

Some states have laws mandating the reporting of elder abuse; others have laws for voluntary reporting of elder abuse. The Elder Abuse and Neglect Act in the state of Illinois, for example, encourages the reporting of elder abuse while also recognizing the right to self-determination of elderly people (that is, as adults, they have the right *not* to report any actions taken against them).[19] If a report is made in good faith in this state, then the health professional cannot be held responsible. Box 7–2 summarizes some basic facts about elder abuse.

Box 7-2. SOME FACTS ABOUT ELDER ABUSE

- Most of the 50 states offer some form of protective services to the abused; however, most such programs are "seriously underfinanced."[20]
- Forty-two of the states have a mandatory reporting feature in their state law.[21]
- Seventy percent of the physicians surveyed in North Carolina and Michigan did not know they were required to report elder abuse.[22]
- In a study of Alabama nurses, 33% of RNs and 40% LPNs seeing elder abuse did not report it. Of the sample of RNs, 57% had seen elder abuse in the past year and 63% had seen it in their career. However, only 29% of the group reporting abuse felt that it had been "handled satisfactorily."[23]
- About 40% of reported cases of elder abuse refused intervention and service.[24]

Gilbert[25] believes that mandatory reporting abuse statutes "reinforce the false idea that old age is automatically accompanied by incompetence." She further notes that "unless it can be shown by clear and convincing evidence that someone age 60 or more lacks the mental capacity to consent or that he or she is a danger to society, he or she is ethically entitled to self-determination." Otherwise, one is treating elderly people just as one would treat children.

Gilbert also identifies the following three ethical dilemmas in reporting elder abuse:

- *Removing harm versus obtaining consent.* In some cases, ethicists believe that if the older person does not want the harm to be reported (thus, the health-care worker cannot secure consent), this overrides the need to remove harm.
- *Preventing harm versus protecting confidentiality.* Again, the promotion of confidentiality is a well-accepted ethical stance. A family member abusing an older person might be protected by confidentiality; however, a nurse doing so might not be, since he or she could harm many others.
- *Promoting benefits versus inflicting no harm (beneficence versus nonmaleficience).* If no service is provided to the older adult who is being abused, more harm than good can result. In Alabama, for example, the reporting of abuse increased 15-fold in the 11-year period since implementation of the Alabama Protective Services Act of 1976. This has simply made "the waiting lists grow longer" when cases are found eligible.

These dilemmas make the reporting of elder abuse a difficult ethical decision for the health-care worker. There is no one easy answer to the problem.

DISCUSSION QUESTION

Put yourself in the place of an older person being abused. Why might you *not* want the abuse to be reported? Does an older person have the right not to have abuse reported? If so, at what point does that no longer hold true? How can you best be an advocate for the abused older patient? Would there ever be cases in which you would be an advocate for the abused older person by *not* reporting abuse?

THE PATIENT OR PRACTITIONER WITH HIV

The risk of a health-care worker's transmitting HIV to a patient is considerably lower than the risk of transmitting other infections, such as hepatitis B, to patients.[26] Similarly, it is difficult for a patient to transmit the virus to a health-care worker. Of course, the risk is increased when procedures become more invasive, as in cardiac catheterization, interventional radiography, nuclear medicine, and ultrasound biopsies.

Many health professionals (a majority of about 58%) appear to believe that patients should know if a health-care worker is HIV-positive before receiving treatment.[27] The Kimberly Bergalis case, in which a young woman died from HIV transmission from her infected dentist, focused on the patient's right to know the HIV status of the health-care provider. The American Medical Association states that physicians should divulge their HIV status "to colleagues" in order to better assess the risk to patients.[28] Different states have different requirements. For example, New York does not require health-care workers to disclose HIV status, relying instead on universal precautions.[29]

The Americans with Disabilities Act protects employees with AIDS against discrimination if they are otherwise qualified. However, Wicher[26] states that if reasonable accommodations cannot be made and the employee poses a risk to patients, that employee can be discharged.

CASE STUDY

THE HIV-POSITIVE COLLEAGUE

Jon Smith has worked in a small community hospital for a long period of time and has become friends with one of the radiologists, Karl Habermass. One day, Karl tells him in confidence that he is HIV-positive.

Jon is faced with a dilemma. Should he report Karl? Does the fact that he is a friend influence the decision in any way? The primary consideration should be whether he believes that harm will come to patients as a result of the HIV status of the radiologist. However, certainly the respect and professional trust he feels for Karl will play a role in the process. These and other arguments for and against reporting are summarized in Table 7–1.

Are radiologic science professionals obligated to work with HIV-positive patients? The short answer to this question is yes. Principle 3 of the ASRT Code of Ethics states: "The Radiologic Technologist delivers patient care and service unrestricted by concerns of personal attributes or the nature of the disease or illness, and without discrimination, regardless of sex, race, creed, religion, or socioeconomic status."[30] A deontologist would thus hold that anyone who is a radiologic science professional must treat HIV-positive and patients with AIDS under all circumstances. An individual who is unwilling to work with such patients should not be a radiologic science professional.

How do some medical imaging professionals feel about caring for HIV-positive patients and patients with AIDS? Table 7–2 summarizes the results of an attitude survey conducted by the author among radiographers, first- and second-year students, and pre-allied health students along with a survey of a group of medical and nursing students.[31] Although this survey was not broad enough to be able to say that it is representative of the entire population, it does show mostly positive attitudes, with some exceptions.

DISCUSSION QUESTION

Many of the questions in Table 7–1 have ethical implications. Do you believe, for example, that professional health-care workers have the right to refuse to work with certain types of patients? If you believe that special hospitals are necessary for patients with AIDS, do you believe that there are other groups that must be segregated? One student, in a discussion session following the survey, stated that he believed that AIDS was a punishment and that even homosexuals who were infected with the virus from a blood transfusion deserved it. Do you agree with this? If not, how would you convince him otherwise?

TABLE 7–1
**ARGUMENTS FOR AND AGAINST REPORTING
HIV-POSITIVE COWORKER**

For Reporting	*Against Reporting*
Patient's right to quality care (beneficence versus maleficence)	Radiologist's right to practice and your confidence in his or her abilities
Right of patient to know	Right of radiologist to confidentiality
State law may mandate reporting	Laws are not always based on sound decisions

TABLE 7-2
ATTITUDES ABOUT AIDS AND AIDS PATIENTS

	Percentage of Yes Responses				
	PAH	RDT1	RDT2	RTs	Currey*
1. If given a choice, would you be willing to treat a patient with AIDS?	73%	85%	58%	72%	60%
2. If given a choice, would you be willing to treat homosexuals?	73%	92%	67%	93%	72%
3. If given a choice, would you be willing to treat IV drug abusers?	63%	85%	67%	93%	73%
4. Would you be willing to perform mouth-to-mouth resuscitation on an AIDS patient?	17%	0%	0%	21%	24%
5. Has your professional education prepared you sufficiently to work safely with AIDS patients?	27%	23%	58%	57%	46%
6. Are you concerned that working with AIDS patients may endanger your health?	50%	100%	83%	86%	71%
7. Should health-care workers have the right to refuse to work with AIDS patients?	83%	76%	75%	57%	54%
8. Should hospitals terminate employees who refuse to treat AIDS patients?	7%	23%	8%	36%	19%
9. Should AIDS patients be treated only in special hospitals and clinics?	30%	46%	33%	43%	29%
10. Homosexuals with AIDS deserve their fate because of their lifestyle.	17%	30%	25%	0%	10%

PHA = pre-allied health; RDT1 = first-year students; RDT2 = second-year students; RTs = radiologic technologists.
*Currey, CJ, Johnson, M, and Ogden, B: Willingness of health-professions students to treat patients with AIDS. Academic Medicine 65(7):472–474, 1990.
SOURCE: Adapted from Dowd,[31] with permission.

THE DYING PATIENT

Death and dying has intrigued philosophers and medical professionals throughout the centuries. In early history, it was accepted that treatment would be terminated in hopeless or severe cases, and that medicine might have a role in hastening the dying process.[32] However, Christianity found itself at odds with such beliefs because of its emphasis on the sanctity of life. As medicine advanced, the possibility of extending life became a reality. Today modern advances in technology have increased attention to the quality of that extended life, and have made names such as Kevorkian, Cruzan, and Quinlan well-known (Box 7–3). Now the "slippery slope" argument has been added to the debate: If one promotes active euthanasia (as practiced by Dr. Jack Kevorkian) in one instance, what prevents its application in others? For example, should seriously deformed children be terminated? The Nazi experiments in the 1940s gave such arguments serious credence.

Box 7–3. ADVANCE MEDICAL DIRECTIVES

Two items have driven the case for advance medical directives (AMDs): the United States Supreme Court decision in *Cruzan v. Director, Missouri Department of Health and the Patient Self-Determination Act,* and part of the Omnibus Budget Reconciliation Act of 1990.[33] The types of advance medical directives are:

- Living Will: A document that expresses a patient's wishes about medical care to be used when a patient is no longer able to make such assertions. Only valid if permitted by state law.
- Natural-Death Act Statutes: Also called a death-with-dignity law, it is a declaration that binds the caregiver to withhold or withdraw life-prolonging treatment.
- Durable Power of Attorney: Given to surrogates who can then make medical decisions for an individual who has become mentally incapacitated.
- Do-Not-Resuscitate Orders (DNRs): An order in the chart to not use life-prolonging treatment such as artificial resuscitation. These provide a number of ethical dilemmas because of their inconsistent execution in hospitals.

CASE STUDY

THE PATIENT'S CHOICE

Sarah Stack is a radiation therapist who has a long-standing relationship with Mr. Smith, who is also a patient. She has known Mr. Smith as a neighbor since childhood, and she was always glad to see him when he arrived for his treatments. Now, however, he is no longer receiving curative treatments; his treatments are for palliation and prolongation of life only. He will probably live 6 months with treatment, but will die relatively soon if he does not continue.

Mr. Smith has decided to not continue with the treatments and to simply let the illness run its course. According to the concepts of autonomy and informed consent, he has the right to do so. However, the paternalistic viewpoint of most medical professionals encourages them to try to convince the patient to continue treatment. A small portion of paternalism in the medical setting is acceptable; however, once the patient understands the consequences, he or she is free to make a decision, even if it seems to be a bad one.

The philosophical analogy lies in an argument proposed by John Stuart Mill.[34] He felt that if a man was about to cross an unsafe bridge, it was an individual's duty to restrain that man long enough to tell him about the danger. If he chose to cross after that, however, he should be allowed to do so.

Mr. Smith's personal physician wants Sarah to convince him to continue with the treatments. She agrees to speak with him, but finds that he understands fully the consequences of his actions and does have grounds for not continuing. Although Sarah disagrees with his reasoning, she believes it is his right to be treated, and does not try to convince him further.

Mr. Smith is asking for passive euthanasia (also called negative euthanasia), in which extraordinary means are not used to prolong life. Positive euthanasia (also called active euthanasia or mercy killing), as advocated by individuals such as Dr. Kevorkian, withdraws life support and/or uses procedures or medications that result in death. In the past, health professionals found it difficult to support either type of euthanasia. This was due to a strictly deontologic or duty-based view of the role of the health professional—a duty to prolong life. Today most health professionals find passive euthanasia acceptable (although they may not support it), but still tend to find active euthanasia objectionable. This is a more teleologic or pragmatic view that accepts the idea that, in some cases, life might not be worth living.

DISCUSSION QUESTION

The movie *Whose Life Is It Anyway* offers an excellent dramatized discussion of passive euthanasia. Watch this movie and discuss the following:

1. Do you believe that patients in their right mind have the right to decline further treatment?
2. How did the health professionals in this movie treat Ken (the patient)? Why did they act this way?

THE PATIENT WITH A DISABILITY

The terms used to describe patients with disabilities have changed over the years. At one time, "handicapped" was an acceptable term, but this is no longer true. The roots of this term come from the beggars who stretched out their caps for handouts. It does not reflect the current status in our society of "people with disabilities," which is the preferred overall term, since it labels them as people first.[35] The term "retarded" is definitely offensive; "developmentally disabled" is the preferred term.

There are many conditions that can lead to disability (Table 7–3). However, not all individuals with these conditions will be disabled. There are a number of special adaptations available today that make individuals with a disability able to perform the tasks of daily living.

People with disabilities may also require special adaptations by the imaging professional. Unger[36] discusses these adaptations. His typology of developmentally disabled patients is shown in Table 7–4.

Although these individuals are protected under a number of laws, such as the Individuals with Disabilities Education Act (PL 102-119) and the

TABLE 7–3
SOME CONDITIONS THAT MAY LEAD TO DISABILITY

Acquired immune deficiency syndrome (AIDS)	Friedrich's ataxia
Arthritis	Guillain-Barré syndrome
Arthrogryposis	Hemiplegia
Blindness	Hydrocephalus
Cerebral palsy	Muscular dystrophy
Cystic fibrosis	Myasthenia gravis
Cerebrovascular accident	Paraplegia
Deafness	Progressive spinal atrophy
Encephalitis	Quadriplegia

Americans with Disabilities Act (ADA), Will[37] has noted that "a multiplication of rights—legally enforceable claims on the attention, actions, and resources of others—can carry us only so far." The way to improve conditions for the disabled, he believes, is to improve the attitudes of the nondisabled.

People with disabilities should be considered a "minority," according to Wertlieb,[38] because they exhibit the following attributes: nonacceptance, stigma, social distance, noncomparability, role strain, negative stereotypes, prejudice and discrimination (often masked, she notes, by an air of protectiveness), and an external locus of control (e.g., a lack of autonomy). Just as Will calls for improvements in attitudes, Wertlieb calls for improvements in knowledge to improve attitudes and reduce what she calls "ambiguous

TABLE 7–4
ADAPTATIONS FOR DEVELOPMENTALLY DISABLED PEOPLE

Type	*Abilities*	*Adaptation for Medical Imagers*
I (lowest level)	Cannot walk, no effective speech, cannot respond appropriately to directions.	Must be lifted to table, positioned, and probably restrained or immobilized. May need nasogastric tube for examinations such as upper GI.
II	Ambulatory; walks alone or unsteadily with help.	Cannot respond to directions, must be positioned, may need restraints.
III	Can walk alone steadily (unless crippling deformity exists), can understand speech.	Can help to position self, may hold still, restraints not usually needed. Types I–III need help changing into gown (in most cases).
IV	Similar to type III, but at a higher level of functioning.	Same as III; can probably change self (but may forget to put gown on after undressing).

SOURCE: Unger.[36]

interaction"—those often uncomfortable interactions we have with individuals we know little about. Recognize that classifications such as Unger's can just as easily be damaging as helpful if we follow them blindly, always seeking to make people fit some preconceived category. For example, use of the term "the disabled" can be seen as a derogatory way to lump people together.[35] Shapiro[39] notes that a number of disabled individuals do not seek medical care because they do not wish to be labeled as "sick." They fear being treated as something less than human by health-care professionals.

The Severely Disabled Newborn

> **DISCUSSION QUESTION**
> One ethical dilemma that confronts the U.S. health-care system is the treatment of severely disabled newborns. Should only those infants who have potential for human relationships be treated, with those whose potential is simply nonexistent or who would be utterly submerged and undeveloped in the mere struggle to survive being allowed to die?[40] Should active euthanasia, the killing of such patients, be acceptable, or should passive euthanasia (e.g., withholding feedings) be allowed?

Imaging professionals such as radiographers and ultrasonographers may be called upon to image patients in the neonatal intensive care unit. Although not directly involved in the ethical decision to treat such a patient, such encounters can be disturbing. Fry-Revere[41] cites a case in which the parents cannot decide whether to approve a series of operations designed to extend the life of a severely disabled newborn or to request only palliative care. Would a hospital bioethics service (if available) be helpful to the nurses and parents in the decision-making process? Will the bioethics service take the needs of the family into consideration?

The French term *anomie* (a, without + *nomos*, law) means "lack of purpose, identity, or ethical values in a person or in a society."[42] Such feelings can occur in health-care workers who are exposed to situations that constantly challenge their ethical values, especially when they are unable to exert any control or influence over the situation. To prevent that from occurring, imaging professionals should clarify their ethical values by answering the following questions:

1. Do I support either active or passive euthanasia?
2. Can I work in an institution where decisions other than the ones I support are followed?

Professionals should recognize that a number of situations are beyond their control. Those who are unable to routinely tolerate such situations may decide to seek employment in settings (e.g., outpatient care) in which they will rarely encounter these ethical challenges.

REFERENCES

1. Verzemnieks, IL, and Nash, D: Ethical issues related to pediatric care. Nurs Clin North Am 19:319–328, 1984.
2. American Academy of Pediatrics, Committee on Pediatric Emergency Care. Consent for medical services for children and adolescents. Pediatrics 92:290–291, 1993.
3. Arizona Revised Statutes section 13-3620.
4. Rhodes, AM: Identifying and reporting child abuse. American Journal of Maternal Child Nursing 12(6):399, 1987.
5. Dowd, SB: Reporting child abuse. Administrative Radiology, 1993, p 63–64.
6. New Jersey Statutes 9.608.10.
7. Alabama Code 26-14-3.
8. Colorado Children's Code Article 19 section 19-10-104.
9. Virginia Code Chapter 12.1 section 63.1-248.3.
10. West Virginia Code section 49-6-A-1.
11. Maryland Family Law Code section 5-901.
12. Oregon Revised Statutes section 418.470.
13. District of Columbia Code 2-1352(c).
14. Wisonsin Statutes section 48.981.
15. Rubinstein v. Baron, 529A 2d 1061 (Superior Court, New Jersey), 1987.
16. Birren, R: Child abuse: Where are we going? NY State J Med 3:133, 1989.
17. Watkins, M: Can you tread this emotional high wire? Balancing elderly people's rights and independence against risks they pose. Professional Nurse 8:604–608, 1993.
18. Niemira, D: Life on the slippery slope: A bedside view of treating incompetent elderly patients. Hastings Cent Rep 23(3):14-17, 1993.
19. Public Act 85-1184; III Revised Statutes Chapter 23, para 6601 et seq.
20. Daniels, RS, Baumhover, LA, and Clark-Daniels, CL: Physicians' mandatory reporting of elder abuse. Gerontologist 29:321–327, 1989.
21. Culhane, C: Federal, state effort in order to prevent elder abuse. American Medical News, July 21, 1989, p 18–19.
22. O'Brien, JG: Elder abuse and the primary care physician. Medical Times 114(2):60–64, 1986.
23. Clark-Daniels, C, Daniels, RS, and Baumhover, LA: The dilemma of elder abuse. Home Healthcare Nurse 8(6):7–12, 1990.
24. O'Malley, TA, Everitt, DE, O'Malley, HC, et al: Identifying and preventing family-medicated abuse and neglect of elderly persons. Ann Intern Med 98:998–1005, 1983.
25. Gilbert, DA: The ethics of mandatory elder abuse reporting statutes. Advances in Nursing Science 8(2):51–62, 1986.
26. Wicher, CP: AIDS and HIV: The dilemma of the health care worker. Journal of Neuroscience Nursing 25:118–123, 1993.
27. Halpren, C, et al: Attitudes toward individuals with HIV: A comparison of medical staff, nurses, and students. AIDS Patient Care 7(5):275–279, 1993.
28. American Medical Association Counsel on Ethical and Traditional Affairs: Ethical issues involved in the growing AIDS crisis. JAMA 259:136, 1988.
29. New York State Department of Health. Policy Statement and Guidelines to Prevent Transmission of HIV and Hepatitis B Through Medical/Dental Procedures. Albany, NY, May 1992.
30. ASRT Code of Ethics. Available from the American Society of Radiologic Technologists, Albuquerque, NM.
31. Dowd, SB: The knowledge and attitudes of radiologic technologists and allied health students regarding AIDS and AIDS patients. The Canadian Journal of Medical Radiation Technology 22:19–22, 1991.
32. Cowley, T, Young, E, and Raffin, TA: Care of the dying: An ethical and historical perspective. Crit Care Med 20:1473–1482, 1992.
33. Darr, K: After Cruzan, hospitals and the right to die. Hospital Topics 69(4):4–6, 1991.

34. Mill, JS: On Liberty: Collected Works of John Stuart Mill. Volume 18. Toronto: University of Toronto Press, 1977.

35. McLaughlin, M: Writing about people with disabilities. The Writer 106:29–30, 1993.

36. Unger, SP: Radiography of persons with developmental disabilities. Radiol Technol 53:481–487, 1982.

37. Will, GF: For the handicapped, rights but no welcome. Hastings Cent Rep 16:5–8, 1986.

38. Wertlieb, EC: Minority group status of the disabled. Human Relations 38:1047–1063, 1985.

39. Shapiro, JP: The health care conundrum. Utne Reader 56 (Mar/Apr):109, 1993.

40. McCormick, RA: To save or let die? JAMA 172:229, 1974.

41. Fry-Revere, S: Ethics consultation: An update on accountability issues. Pediatric Nursing 20:95–98, 1994.

42. Webster's New World Dictionary, Second College Edition. New York: Simon and Schuster, 1980.

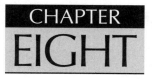

CHAPTER
EIGHT

Charting and Documentation

Bettye G. Wilson, MEd, RT(R)(CT), RDMS

Traditionally, education in the medical imaging professions has not promoted the importance of charting and documentation. In the late 1960s, charts accompanying the patient to the radiology department were largely considered of interest only to the radiologists. Institutions of education in medical imaging, while acknowledging the chart as a vital and integral part of the patient record, failed to educate students on the hows and whens of charting and documentation.

In the mid-1970s, with the addition of computed tomography (CT) and medical ultrasound to many diagnostic radiology departments, charts and medical records began to receive more attention from practitioners. The position of radiology nurse was widely introduced at this time, and the job of charting and documentation in radiology was largely left to these nurses. However, because the majority of radiology nurses had little radiographic procedural knowledge, information retrieval and the entering of pertinent information into the patient's chart were often lacking.

In the late 1970s, more medical imaging professionals began to retrieve vital information from and enter pertinent information into the patient chart. More often than not, these professionals were not provided with adequate instruction on why charting and documentation are necessary, when charting and documentation are required, or how charting and documentation should be accomplished.

119

This chapter provides the reader with information as to why charting and documentation in medical imaging are necessary, when charting and documentation should be done, and how to chart or document. Further, the ethics and legalities of charting and documentation are discussed.

OBJECTIVES

At the end of this chapter, the reader will be able to:

- Define the terms charting and documenting
- List the components of the medical chart
- List reasons why prompt, accurate charting is necessary
- Describe areas of the patient chart where information concerning allergies, current history, symptomology and status, laboratory reports, medications, physician orders, and medical imaging reports may be located
- List specific areas of medical imaging that should always be documented

WHAT ARE CHARTING AND DOCUMENTATION?

Charting can be described simply as the recording of information and observations regarding patient care on the written record, that is, the patient's chart. In the broadest sense, documentation means the recording of any information affecting the care of the patient. In medical imaging departments, not all documentation is done in the patient's chart. For example, the documentation of the last menstrual period (LMP) of a female patient about to undergo an abdominal fluoroscopic procedure may be recorded on the examination request form.

Both charting and documenting are written communication tools that provide comprehensive medical information on an individual patient basis.[1] The patient's medical record is a legal document, and it is admissible in litigation as evidence of the care given the patient and the standards under which that care was provided.[2] The accuracy and clarity of the information in the patient's medical record are important to the facility providing the patient's care, to the provider of that care, and to the patient.[3]

Many medical lawsuits may take years to be heard in court. Chances are that time will have dulled the memories of those involved, and the medical record may be the only accurate recollection and defense of past actions. Therefore, it is imperative that medical records pertinent to the case be complete and accurate at the time they are written.

MEDICAL MALPRACTICE LITIGATION AND DOCUMENTATION

Malpractice in medicine is defined as injurious or unprofessional treatment of a patient. Suits for malpractice are not limited to treatment by physicians.

Medical imaging professionals as well as other health-care providers can be sued for malpractice. Also, the legal definition of malpractice has been expanded to include neglect. The focus of medical malpractice is usually restricted to four areas: duty, breach of duty, causation, and damage. The sequence of events in medical malpractice occur as follows:

Duty

It must be proven that the medical professional involved has a duty to the patient. In medical imaging this occurs when the medical imaging professional and patient relationship is established (i.e., as late as when the procedure is actually performed or as early as when you introduce yourself to the patient, informing him or her that you will be the person performing the exam). The medical imaging professional's duty to the patient is to provide quality patient care that follows appropriate professional standards.

Breach of Duty

It must be ascertained that the provider has breached the duty owed the patient. In other words, have you as a medical imaging professional failed to provide the patient with the standard of care sanctioned by your profession and exhibited by the majority of practitioners of the profession? A question that may be posed to determine if a breach of duty has occurred might be: How would a reasonable, prudent medical imaging professional with comparable education, training, and experience have acted in the same circumstances or similar ones? Documentation of what was done, how it was done, when it was done, and who did it is critical in making a breach of duty determination.

Causation and Damage

Causation and damage is the determination, after establishing that a breach of duty has occurred, that the breach of duty caused injury (damage) to the patient. While causation is the one area of malpractice most difficult to establish,[2] proper documentation can be instrumental in refuting a claim of malpractice.

The legal medical record does not consist only of the patient's chart. Of particular interest to those in the medical imaging professions is the inclusion of radiographic images, including CT, magnetic resonance imaging (MRI), and ultrasound. These must also exhibit characteristic good record-keeping practices as defined under federal and state laws, accreditation agency parameters, institutional policy and procedure, and departmental protocol.

STANDARDS FOR DOCUMENTATION

What is documented concerning patient care varies from facility to facility, based primarily on the overall needs of each facility. However, state and federal laws and accreditation commissions like the Joint Commission on the Accreditation of Healthcare Organizations (JCAHO) prescribe minimum requirements for the contents of medical records.

Outpatient centers such as ambulatory surgery centers and free-standing medical imaging centers may require different documentation than do their inpatient counterparts. Long-term care facilities, while more akin to hospitals than outpatient centers, may also require different documentation. In all types of medical facilities, however, accurate, complete health-care service records are essential for documenting quality patient care. Although medical records may have important legal implications, they are first and foremost clinical communication tools that should be documented carefully.[2] Anyone who enters data into the patient record should realize the importance of keeping an accurate, objective, and all-inclusive document.[3]

According to the JCAHO, the leading accreditation body for hospitals, a medical record "contains sufficient information to identify the patient, support the diagnosis, justify the treatment, document the course and results, and promote continuity of care among health care providers."[4] Medicare legislation concerning medical record documentation guidelines states that "the hospital medical record must contain information to justify the admission and continued hospitalization, support the diagnosis, and describe the patient's progress and response to the medication and services."[5] Health-care insurance companies require that medical records contain sufficient information to support the diagnosis for reimbursement purposes under the diagnosis-related groups (DRGs) and the prospective payment system (PPS) implemented by the federal government in 1983. The preceding are just a few of the required content standards for medical records. Maintaining complete and accurate records is essential for quality patient care, clinical decision making, and financial reimbursement by private insurance companies and state and federal medical insurance programs.

While medical records or health information management departments are generally responsible for overseeing patient records, correct and sufficient patient data entry into the medical record is the job of everyone rendering direct patient care. Health-care providers in any facility must be familiar with the medical record format of that facility. Generally, most inpatient facilities follow the standards for inpatient medical records prescribed by the JCAHO. These standards include, but are not limited to, the following data:

- Patient identification information
- Medical history
- Psychosocial needs summary
- Physical examination report

- Conclusion or impression statement on the admission history and physical examination (H & P)
- Treatment plan
- Diagnostic and therapeutic orders
- Evidence of informed consent for appropriate procedures
- Clinical observations, which include the results of therapy
- Progress notes
- Consultation reports
- Reports of surgical and invasive procedures; tests and their results
- Reports from diagnostic and therapeutic procedures
- Records regarding the donation or receipt of implants or transplants
- Final diagnosis or diagnoses
- Conclusions at termination of hospitalization
- Discharge summary and clinical résumés
- Discharge information provided to the patient or patient's family members
- Results of postmortem examination if performed.[4]

DISCUSSION QUESTION

From the preceding list of JCAHO Standards, can you name and locate areas of the medical record where the following would be charted?

1. Request for an intravenous urogram (IVU)
2. Consent form for an IVU
3. Report from IVU

RECORDING IN THE MEDICAL RECORD

Since the medical record is a legal written communication tool used to provide a record of a coordinated approach to the diagnosis and treatment of the individual patient, certain criteria for the recording of information in that record must be strictly adhered to. Table 8–1 list the dos and don'ts of recording information in the medical record.

The information provided in Table 8–1 is basically self-explanatory. However, some areas may raise a few questions. For example, some may ask why the time of the entry should be written in military time. The reason is that military time does not require that A.M. or P.M. be written, therefore no confusion is created if A.M. or P.M. is not included. Military time equivalents for standard A.M. and P.M. designations are listed in Table 8–2. When designating minutes in military time, simply add the minutes after the hour designation. For example: If the standard time notation would be 7:05 A.M., the military time equivalent is 0705. Rarely is it necessary to chart time using

TABLE 8–1
RECORDING INFORMATION IN THE MEDICAL RECORD

Do	Don't
1. Write legibly.	1. Write in pencil.
2. Write in ink.	2. Block out or erase entries.
3. Use correct spelling and standard medical abbreviations.	3. Enter unnecessary details.
4. Write accurate information: correct and precise.	4. Include critical comments about the patient or other health-care professionals.
5. Keep the information concise.	5. Leave blank spaces in your notes.
6. Provide thorough entries.	6. Use improper abbreviations.
7. Begin each entry with the date and time (military) of the entry.	7. Record information for someone else.
8. Record information as it occurs.	8. Divulge information concerning the patient; this information is confidential.
9. Keep information confidential.	9. Use initials when signing your name.
10. Sign each entry with *your* name and title.	

TABLE 8–2
MILITARY TIME EQUIVALENTS FOR STANDARD TIME NOTATIONS

Standard Time Notation	Military Time Equivalent
1:00 A.M.	0100
2:00 A.M.	0200
3:00 A.M.	0300
4:00 A.M.	0400
5:00 A.M.	0500
6:00 A.M.	0600
7:00 A.M.	0700
8:00 A.M.	0800
9:00 A.M.	0900
10:00 A.M.	1000
11:00 A.M.	1100
12:00 noon	1200
1:00 P.M.	1300
2:00 P.M.	1400
3:00 P.M.	1500
4:00 P.M.	1600
5:00 P.M.	1700
6:00 P.M.	1800
7:00 P.M.	1900
8:00 P.M.	2000
9:00 P.M.	2100
10:00 P.M.	2200
11:00 P.M.	2300
12:00 midnight	2400

seconds. If it is necessary to do so, however, use a colon and the number of seconds after the minute notation. Example: 7:05 A.M. and 30 seconds would be 705:30 A.M. in standard time and 0705:30 in military time.

Writing only in ink in the medical record lends permanence to that record. Many institutions request that only black ink be used when charting and may also specifically prohibit the use of red ink. Others may allow both blue and black ink. A review of the health information management (medical records) policies and procedures at your facility should clearly define what is acceptable. Erasures, blocked-out entries, and blank spaces are unacceptable. If an error is made in the patient's chart, it should be corrected only by the person who made the error as soon as the error is discovered. The person making the error draws a line through the error, documents that an error has occurred by writing an explanation near it, writes in the correct information, and then dates and signs the correction[6] (Fig. 8–1).

Note that Figure 8–1 also demonstrates that any blank spaces should be filled with lines. And remember, do not use correction fluid or otherwise block out entries so that they cannot be read. It is essential that the original entry be legible.

Late entries into the medical record should be avoided. Late and altered entries may arouse suspicion in the event of malpractice litigation. These types of entries may suggest to the courts that other alterations to the record have also occurred. The validity of the entire medical record may be seriously compromised because of one late or altered entry.

If your facility has a protocol for making late entries into the medical record, follow that protocol when a late entry must be made. If no late-entry protocol has been established by your facility, the following steps may be used:

1. Add the entry to the first available line on the documentation form where you should make your entry (progress notes, nurse's notes, medication administration, etc.).
2. Clearly label the entry "late entry." This will indicate that you know that the entry is out of sequence.

7/21/96	0900	~~Ba. enema~~ complete. pt. may resume diet as ordered by
		physician. ———————————— *Bettye Wilson, R7 (R)*
7/21/96	0902	*Ba. swallow complete. pt. may resume diet as ordered*
		by physician. ———————————— *Bettye Wilson, R7 (R)*

FIGURE 8–1. Example of correct method of recording an error in documentation.

3. Record the time and date of the entry.
4. In the body of your entry, record the time and date that the entry should have been made.
5. Sign your entry.[2]

Never include critical comments about the patient or other health-care professionals in your documentation. If this information is admitted in a court of law, it can be used to support claims of negligence or inadequate care. Also, critical comments present evidence of a disjointed health-care team when the team should provide a continuum of quality care. Finally, critical comments made by an individual may require that individual to defend them in court.

Only standard and acceptable abbreviations and symbols should be used when charting. Everyone who documents patient care should become familiar with these symbols and abbreviations. Nursing service and medical information management departments are good sources for locating this information. In-service education can also be a valuable source of information on charting and documentation as well as on other departmental and hospital policies and procedures.

Legally, if something is not charted or otherwise documented, it has not been done. Nothing can be proved if no written record exists. Many juries have heard attorneys say "not charted, not done." Only accurate, concise, and careful documentation can substantiate events concerning patient care.

ETHICAL ISSUES IN CHARTING AND DOCUMENTATION

The legal implications of proper charting and documentation are readily identifiable, but the ethical issues are just as important. Some of the ethical issues of charting and documentation also have legal implications. Medical ethics has long been a part of medical practice. The 1960s, however, ushered in an era in which ethical problems in health care have increased in both complexity and quantity.[2]

Ethical questions in charting and documentation most often involve situations surrounding decisions regarding informed consent and patient confidentiality. Informed consent in its truest form can be obtained only by the physician because it should include, at the minimum, information on the following:

1. An explanation of the procedure
2. Benefits of having the procedure performed
3. What knowledge can be derived from the procedure
4. What could happen if the procedure is not performed
5. What risks are associated with the procedure
6. What alternatives there are to the proposed procedure

The education and experience of the physician qualifies him or her, under the law, as the only person able to factually and fully answer the questions that surround informed consent.[2]

However, many professionals in health care are aware that, in practice, consent for a medical procedure may be obtained by nurses or other health-care providers. Some of the ethical principles that may be compromised when health-care professionals other than physicians obtain consent are veracity (truth telling); autonomy (the right of the patient to information that will enable the patient to determine what is best for him or her); and fidelity (being faithful to the patient's expectations of care). Unless specific hospital policies and procedures allow health-care professionals other than physicians to obtain informed consent, only the physician should undertake this task.

Patient confidentiality is a requirement of every health-care professional. No information concerning the patient should be divulged to any person without a professional need to know—information should be shared only with those directly involved in that patient's care.

The American Hospital Association's "A Patient's Bill of Rights" states that "the patient has the right to expect that all communications and records pertaining to his care be treated as confidential." Everyone involved in patient care is obligated to uphold this right. Conversations in public places regarding patients should be avoided. "Elevator talk" about patients and other health-care professionals has provided fodder for lawsuits in too many instances. Remember, you never know who knows whom. Also, do not discuss or release patient information to unauthorized individuals without the written consent of the patient. The ethical principles of nonmaleficence (not doing harm), beneficence (doing good), and fidelity (faithfulness to the patient's expectations) are involved in patient confidentiality.

Under certain conditions, the law requires that confidential information regarding the patient be disclosed. These situations may include:

1. Civil cases
2. Criminal cases
3. Suspected nonaccidental trauma (child abuse)
4. Matters of public health and safety

Even when required to disclose confidential, privileged information, health-care professionals should safeguard as much information as they can. Only subpoenaed information should be disclosed.

Access patient information only when it is necessary for you to perform your job. Just because you have access to an individual's record does not mean you should abuse that privilege. For example, is it really necessary for you to look into your neighbor's chart to see why he or she is in the hospital if you are not involved in his or her care?

PROCEDURES AND FORMS IN MEDICAL IMAGING DOCUMENTATION

Educational programs in medical imaging and therapy have largely ignored the structured teaching of charting and documentation, preferring instead that students learn what to do in the clinical setting or providing bits and pieces in other structured courses. Perhaps it is time to recognize that, as members of the health-care team, medical imaging professionals should be as skilled in the art of charting and documentation as they are in the services they provide.

Critical areas of documentation in medical imaging and therapy include the following:

1. Pertinent patient history, including vital signs
2. Technical variables
3. Contrast media or radiopharmaceutical administration
4. Pre- and postprocedure directions
5. Name and credentials of personnel involved in the procedure
6. Radiographic interpretation of findings from the procedure by the radiologist, sonologist,* cardiologist, or other physician[3]
7. Procedure consent forms
8. Patient education
9. Incident reports
10. Changes in patient status
11. Reactions to contrast media administration and what steps, if any, were taken to treat the reaction
12. Documentation of additional radiation protection when required, such as in pregnant patients whose doctors have decided that the performance of a radiographic procedure is absolutely necessary even though the patient is pregnant
13. The date of the last menstrual period (LMP), as attested to by the patient, of any female patient about to undergo a procedure in which ionizing radiation will be delivered to the abdominal or pelvic region

As charting and documentation procedures vary from facility to facility, it is imperative that imaging professionals become familiar with the requirements for charting and documentation at their facility.[7]

To assess the variations in charting and documentation among facilities, this author conducted a telephone survey. Diagnostic radiology, ultrasound, and CT departments in eight hospitals were contacted. The hospitals ranged in size from slightly less than 200 beds to 750 beds.

Surprisingly, the area of diagnostic radiology reported documenting, in

---

* Sonologist—physician, radiologist or other, whose speciality area is ultrasonography.

some fashion, more than the other areas (8 of 8). CT was next with 6 of the 8 facilities reporting charting, while ultrasound came in last with 5 of 8 reporting charting. All diagnostic radiology departments documented on the imaging procedure requisition as well as in the patient's chart. CT documented more in the patient's chart (5 of 6) than on the requisition, and ultrasound reported documenting more in the patient's chart (4 of 5). Progress notes were most often cited as the area of the patient's chart used by medical imaging professionals for documentation purposes (12 of 14), while the nurse's notes were largely ignored as was the medication record.

Critical information in medical imaging and therapy should be documented on the patient history and physical (H&P) form, the medical imaging requisition form, and the patient's chart.

Patient History and Physical Form

The H&P, which generally contains patient identification and demographic information, medical history, and current symptomology and tentative diagnosis, should include a section where medical imaging professionals can write information concerning the patient in relation to the procedure. This should be the area where responses to questions about the LMP or pregnancy of a female patient are recorded. This is also the area where a form signed by female patients considered still in the gene pool should be placed. These forms, when required by the medical imaging department or facility, should inform the patient of the risks attributed to radiation exposure of the fetus during pregnancy, especially during the first trimester, when organogenesis is occurring and the fetus is most sensitive to the effects of radiation.

Patient allergies should be "flagged" on the front of the patient's chart and documented on the H&P form. If the medical imaging professional discovers that the patient has an allergy that is not noted on the chart, he or she should place that information in the H&P comment or note section.

Medical Imaging Requisition Form

The recording of technical information is often seen as applicable only to staff radiographers. But other medical imaging professionals such as ultrasonographers, CT technologists, interventional technologists, and magnetic resonance technologists should also record this information. The information can be recorded on the procedure requisition (request) form and on the patient's chart. Before recording the information on the request form only, make sure that the original request is placed in the patient's permanent medical record (chart) or at least that a copy is filed with the hard copy images.

Radiographers should document the kilovoltage peak (kVp) and the milliamperage (mA) and time (seconds) or milliamperage per second (mA × time = mAs). If the procedure used was fluoroscopy, the amount of fluoro on-time should also be recorded. When using automatic exposure control (AEC), the mA readout for each exposure should be recorded. The number of radiographs taken should also be recorded, along with the number of repeats made, if required by departmental procedure. CT technologists may want to record the same information, substituting images filmed for radiographs taken, since multiple images may appear on one film in CT. Even though technical information is usually automatically recorded on the hard copy, ultrasonographers may want to document information such as transducer used and depth and gain settings.

Patient's Chart

Information about the medical imaging procedure, including contrast medium or radiopharmaceutical administration, pre- and postprocedure directions, and names and credentials of persons performing the procedure, should be recorded in the patient's chart on either the medication record, nurses' notes, or progress report. Since contrast agents and radiopharmaceuticals are considered drugs, information concerning their administration should be documented on the medication record. This documentation should consist of the date and time, mode of administration (such as IV or oral), name of contrast agent, and amount administered. The person administering the contrast should sign the documentation and provide his or her credentials. If a physician administers the contrast agent or radiopharmaceutical, the medical imaging professional can chart the information for the physician as shown in Figure 8–2.

All drugs given to the patient in the medical imaging department should be documented. These may include, but are not limited to, the following:

- Glucagon for intestinal spasm
- Valium for relief of anxiety
- Benedryl for mild contrast reactions
- IV fluid if the original bag emptied while the patient was in the imaging department

Remember that barium sulfate suspensions such as E-Z CAT and Oral Hy-

| 7/6/96 | 0900 | 100cc of Renografin 60 was administered I.V. by |
| | | radiologist Dr. Ben Pervis. ——— Bettye Wilson, R7 (R) |

FIGURE 8–2. Example of proper documentation of medication administration (administered by physician).

paque are also considered drugs and should be charted as such. The documentation of drugs given to the patient is important because:

1. Adverse reactions may occur.
2. The administration of one drug may contraindicate the administration of another.
3. When a patient has an I & O (intake and output) order, everything that is taken into the patient's body must be recorded.
4. Accreditation bodies such as the JCAHO require the documentation of drugs.
5. Reimbursement by insurance companies and by Medicaid and Medicare hinges on accurate and complete documentation of services provided to the patient.

Adverse reactions to the administration of contrast agents should be documented on the nurse's notes or the progress report. These same forms may also be used to document change in a patient's status while the patient is in the care of the medical imaging professional. For example, if a patient who is alert and well oriented before a procedure becomes confused after the procedure, the radiologist or another physician should be summoned. The change in patient status and the notification of the radiologist or other physician should be documented in the patient's chart.

PATIENT EDUCATION

Patient education is an important responsibility of medical imaging professionals. It is often performed as a part of the introduction protocol between the medical imaging professional and the patient. It is usually so routine that we are not conscious of doing it. However, the education of the patient about the medical imaging procedure to be performed should be documented, especially when it is more involved than a routine chest examination or examination of an extremity. Good communication between the medical imaging professional and the patient is crucial to the performance of a high-quality diagnostic procedure. The more a patient knows about a procedure, the more he or she feels in control of the situation. This supports the patient's need to feel autonomous.

> **DISCUSSION QUESTION**
> Refer to the codes of ethics or conduct in Chapter 3. Are there specific areas in any or all of them that address patient education? Discuss the similarities and differences in each of the codes in regard to patient education.

A procedure that requires IV contrast media or carries potential risks requires patient consent. It is the responsibility of the imaging professional to make sure that this consent is in the patient's chart *before* the patient is premedicated for a procedure that requires premedication or before a procedure that does not require premedication actually begins. This form should be specific to the examination being performed. It should be dated, signed by the patient, and witnessed. The person signing the document as the "witness" can be another health care provider, a family member, or even a visitor. The witness's signature attests only to the fact that the witness saw the person sign the consent form.

Any questions the patient has about the procedure itself may be answered by the medical imaging professional. However, if questions pertain to medical or surgical issues, the patient should be referred to the physician.

INCIDENT REPORTS

Serious incidents involving patients are not common in medical imaging departments, but they do occur. Facilities normally have specific protocols for the reporting of such incidents. These protocols may incorporate state requirements. Medical imaging departments may also have specific guidelines for reporting an incident. There are usually incident report forms of some type to be filled out. Incident reports should include the following information:

1. What happened to the patient
2. The time it happened
3. Where it happened
4. Who and what was involved in the incident
5. Who witnessed or was present when it happened
6. The outcome of the incident
7. What actions were necessary[8]

Incident report forms should not be included in the patient's medical record unless the state requires their inclusion. No reference to the report should be made in the chart either.[3] Incident reports are invaluable to a medical facility if further treatment for injury caused by the incident is needed or if the incident goes to litigation. A clear and factual written report is required for substantiation of the facts.

Incident reports help facilities improve patient care. By reviewing the reports to see how the incident could have been avoided, the offices of risk management, quality assurance, and safety can use the information to educate practitioners and form policies and procedures to avoid a recurrence of the same type of incident.

MEDICAL IMAGES AS RECORDS

It has long been established that radiographs are a part of the medicolegal record of the patient. However, so are ultrasound and magnetic resonance images, along with any computer storage media of these images. These images are the property of the institution in which they were created and do not belong to the patient.

All medical imaging receptors should include areas for certain information, including but not limited to the following:

1. Patient's name
2. Name of the institution
3. Patient's age and/or birthdate
4. Patient's medical record number or medical imaging file number
5. Date of procedure
6. Type of procedure requested
7. Initials of the person performing the procedure

This information may be directly imbedded in the image receptor for radiographs or placed on ultrasound, CT, or MRI images digitally. The information legalizes the images as specifically those of a certain patient.

Only images of high technical quality should be included in the patient's medical imaging record. All other images should be discarded. Some facilities have spaces for documentation of the number of images made and the number of discarded images on the imaging procedure requisition form.

The medical image should, in the case of radiographs, have anatomical side markers radiographed directly onto the image receptor at the time the image is made. Some of these markers include the initials of the person performing the exam. In ultrasound, CT, MRI, and nuclear medicine, patient orientation or anatomical side denotation is digitally placed on the image.

Although state requirements vary, medical images are generally stored for a period of 5 to 7 years for adult patients, and 1 to 7 years after the age of majority (18–21 years) for minors.[7] Some facilities keep current medical imaging records in-house for a period of time and then transfer the records to long-term storage. The records in long-term storage can be easily retrieved if necessary. As with all medical records, storage should be secure. Most medical imaging departments have film libraries specifically for this purpose.

DOCUMENTING RADIATION PROTECTION

The use of ionizing radiation for the production of medical images leading to the diagnosis of illness and disease is more than 100 years old. In the hands of educationally prepared, qualified professionals, its use poses limited hazards. The educational standards for radiologic science professionals ensure that students who attend accredited institutions receive proper instruction in the practice of radiation science and in radiation protection. Documentation of that instruction is housed in the student record at the educational institution.

Most radiographic equipment in use today employs automatic collimation of the x-ray beam. If preventive maintenance, including calibration of the equipment, is routinely performed, the imaging professionals operating the equipment and the patients on whom the equipment is used can be assured that the equipment will not cause them to receive excess radiation. Documentation of equipment maintenance and calibration should be on file in the medical imaging department.

Repeat analysis performed by quality assurance technologists in the imaging department is another means of assessing whether patients are being subjected to more radiation exposure than necessary. Departments should use this information to determine whether repeat rates exceed the acceptable range according to departmental and facility standards. Repeat analysis records should also be stored in the department.

Medical imaging professionals who use ionizing radiation in everyday practice must be diligent in practicing radiation protection for their patients and themselves. The pregnant patient who must be radiographed probably promotes the greatest concern among medical imaging professionals. Remember, if a pregnant patient must be radiographed, use additional radiation protection measures and document, document, document. The progress report form or nurse's notes in the patient's medical chart and the imaging procedure request form can all be used to document this information. A medical release form for the patient who is pregnant may be available in some facilities. This form should educate the patient as to the risks involved in exposing the fetus to ionizing radiation in utero. If the form is used, it should be signed, dated, witnessed, and forwarded through the appropriate channels. Legally, if it's not documented, it was not done.

CONCLUSION

This chapter could not cover every minute aspect of documentation for medical imaging professionals. The author's intent is to facilitate an understanding of the elements of proper charting and documentation and to define the ethical and legal challenges of documentation and charting in the patient care environment. Medical imaging professionals, as invaluable members of the health-care team, pride themselves in the delivery of quality patient care. Legally, if it wasn't charted, it wasn't done. Ethically, if it was not documented accurately and properly, the patient is deprived of certain aspects of quality care. Charting and documentation should be performed with the same high-quality standards as you place on your imaging expertise.

REFERENCES

1. Kowalczy, K, and Donnett, K: Integrated Patient Care for the Imaging Professional. Philadelphia, Mosby-Year Book, 1996.
2. Norris, J: Mastering Documentation. Springhouse, PA, Springhouse Corporation, 1995.

3. Obergfell, A: Law and Ethics in Diagnostic Imaging and Therapeutic Radiology. Philadelphia, WB Saunders, 1996.
4. Comprehensive Accreditation Manual for Hospitals, Oakbrook Terrace, Ill., Joint Commission on Accreditation of Health Care Organizations, 1996.
5. Grostick, S, and Hamer, J: Health Records and Alabama Law, ed 3. Montgomery, Al, Alabama Association of Health Information Management, 1996.
6. Adler, A, and Carlton, R: Introduction to Radiography and Patient Care. Philadelphia, WB Saunders, 1994.
7. Ehrlich, R, and McCloskey, R: Patient Care in Radiography, ed 4. Philadelphia, Mosby-Year Book, 1993.
8. Culmer, P: Chaeney's Care of the Patient in Diagnostic Radiography, ed 7. Oxford, England: Blackwell Science, 1995.

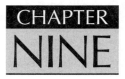

Basic Concepts of Medical Law

Sharon B. Barnes, MPH, ARRT(R)
Steven B. Dowd, EdD, ARRT(R)
Jane Faulkner Evans, JD, ARRT(R)(NMT)

Laws play an important role in the practice of medicine and in the allied health professions. This chapter is designed to help the medical imaging professional understand the law. It defines legal terms and encourages an understanding of responsibility under the law.

Laws are the body of rules, regulations, and guidelines that govern conduct in society to protect the health, safety, and welfare of its citizens. The basis of all types of law is natural law; that is, those actions that are innately correct, such as punishment for murder or theft. Different societies have developed similar fundamental rules based on natural law.

Simple societies require few laws. As society becomes more complex, more laws are necessary to regulate behavior. Complex institutions, such as those devoted to health care, are heavily regulated to ensure the safety of participants (patients) and the accountability of providers (physicians, workers, and administrators). Although law may seem burdensome, its purpose is to promote the common good of society.

Law and ethics are not identical. Although law should represent the ethics of a society, it may not because of special interests. Ethics, especially personal or professional ethics and ethical codes, focus on ideal rather than acceptable or "reasonable" behavior. The law may be much more pragmatic in its view of human behavior.

OBJECTIVES

At the end of this chapter, the reader will be able to:

- Give the reason and rationale for law
- List the sources of law
- Describe the basic sequence of events in a trial
- Differentiate between civil and criminal liability
- Define relevant legal doctrines
- List torts relevant to health-care professionals
- Give examples of actions that may lead to tort charges against those in health care

ESTABLISHMENT OF LAW

Law is a complex concept developed over time to reflect the values of a society. But, as with all complex concepts, there are basic underpinnings for law. Some of these underpinnings are discussed in the following paragraphs.

Concern for Justice and Fairness

Law exists so that the rights of an individual or group cannot be encroached upon by another individual or group. Law (especially as developed by legislators) may, however, be influenced by special interests. This may be unavoidable as long as money is a driving force for humankind.

Dynamic Nature of Law

Society is not static; it is dynamic and always changing. Therefore laws should be able to be changed to meet society's needs. Because of rapid changes in society, law must be flexible enough to meet the needs of new situations.

Ensuring Similar Standards of Performance

All individuals are not held to identical standards; however, those with similar education and training or performing the same job should follow the same guidelines. In cases of tort-law, which includes negligence, the law is based on what reasonable and prudent persons would do in similar circumstances.

Individual Rights and Responsibilities

All individuals have basic rights and responsibilities in each society. In the United States, we believe strongly in the rights of the individual; however, the more rights an individual claims, the greater the responsibility. If responsibilities are not met, the law can restrict the individual's rights.

The four areas described above help guide the establishment of law, but who makes the law? Law does not come from a single source but rather from a variety of sources.

SOURCES OF LAW

Statutory Law

Statutory law is established and enforced by federal, state, and local legislators in response to perceived needs for social regulation. The courts decide how statutory law applies to situations deemed to be the subject of the statute. For example, the court will decide whether certain actions by an individual are actually discriminatory in situations in which discrimination is prohibited by law (such as college admissions).

Administrative Law

Although administrative laws may have the legislature or executive branch as their source, they are issued and enforced by an administrative body on the authority of the legislature or executive branch. Examples of administrative agencies at the federal level that influence health care are the Department of Health and Human Services, the Public Health Service, and the National Labor Relations Board. At the state level, licensure boards and departments of public health are examples of administrative agencies.

Common Law

Common law (or case law) is that body of law and juristic theory originated, developed, and formulated as an outgrowth of English common law. It is the very foundation of American jurisprudence.

Two important principles in common law are *res judicata,* "the thing is decided," and *stare decisis,* "let the decision stand." These principles provide for the resolution of similar or identical legal disputes based on the decisions made in previous cases. These previous cases are precedents. However, the decisions made in these cases are not absolute. Different decisions may be made and new precedents set as a result of changes in societal needs or technology.

Constitutional Law

Formal bodies typically establish themselves through a compact or master plan known as a constitution. The root of law in the United States is the

Constitution of the United States. The federal courts are the final authority in determining the conformity of all laws to the basis of law, the Constitution.

Many of the amendments to the Constitution are relevant to the practice of health care. The First Amendment, for example, establishes freedom of religion, as well as freedom of speech and the right to assembly. For example, this allows nurses who oppose abortion on religious grounds to request alternative assignments if they work in a hospital that performs abortions. The 14th Amendment to the Constitution guarantees each citizen of the United States equal protection of the law. The right to privacy and the right to due process are examples of protections guaranteed by the 14th Amendment.

Privacy and the Abortion Issue

The right to privacy under the 14th Amendment has been interpreted by the Supreme Court to include a woman's right to abortion.[1] This has become a very sensitive issue in health care and politics. Abortion is the medical termination of pregnancy, either elective (by choice) or therapeutic (to save the mother's life). Since the 1973 landmark U.S. Supreme Court case, *Roe v Wade*,[2] every woman has had the legal right to an elective abortion during the first 3 months (called the first trimester) of pregnancy.

Abortion has special implications for medical imaging professionals, specifically sonographers, through the action of wrongful birth suits.[3] Wrongful birth lawsuits are claims against a physician, department, or hospital brought by the parents of a baby born physically or mentally impaired when the parents were not informed of the potential for defect. The parents may believe that they would have avoided conception or terminated the pregnancy if they had been properly advised of the risks and/or the existence of birth defects in the child. Classic cases of wrongful birth typically have involved exposure to rubella. In *Smith v Cote*,[4] a physician failed to test a pregnant woman in a timely fashion for exposure to rubella; in *Proffitt v Bartolo*,[5] a physician failed to interpret a rubella test properly during the first trimester, thereby precluding the option of abortion.

Before so-called abortion on demand, courts would not hear wrongful birth suits, as the outcome (birth) was not preventable by legal means. Most courts still refuse to allow these cases unless a statute expressly authorizes them. California, Illinois, Indiana, New Jersey, and Washington authorize cases only for special damages, such as the extraordinary expenses of the child's illness.

Abortion will continue to be a volatile topic in health care since the U.S. population is so divided on the issue. The Supreme Court has paved the way recently for states to assume greater responsibility in deciding parameters for obtaining abortions. As the law changes, one can expect to see legal challenges as well.

DISCUSSION QUESTION

Unlike most medical imaging professionals, sonographers are often responsible for some basic screening or diagnosis of the image. In one lawsuit, the sonographer told a mother while scanning that her baby was "waving at her." The child was born without limbs. What are some of the implications of assuming this role of diagnosis, especially since many sonographers are trained on the job?

Due Process

Another constitutional guarantee that has special implications for health care, especially education, is due process, which is an outgrowth of the 14th Amendment as interpreted by the courts. Due process has two basic elements.

1. A substantive element, which defines and regulates the rights of citizens and the circumstances under which the state may restrict those rights
2. A procedural element, which requires that a citizen have an opportunity to refute any attempts by government or an entity such as a school to deprive the citizen of substantive rights[6]

A student dismissed from an educational program can lose the right to liberty or property and may not be able to work as a practitioner in that discipline. In the case of *Horowitz v Board of Curators of the University of Missouri,*[7] a medical student was properly dismissed from a medical school because she lacked the appropriate clinical skills. She was fully informed of the potential dismissal. In the case of *Regents of University of Michigan v Ewing,*[8] a medical student was found to have been deprived of his property rights under the 14th Amendment because he was the only student not allowed to retake a test. However, the Supreme Court ruled in favor of the school on appeal because it was found that the decision was based on the student's poor academic record, even though other students also had poor academic records and were allowed to retake the exam.

DISCUSSION QUESTION

Find the due process procedure for your school (all accredited programs have one). Discuss also the procedures used to inform students of "unsatisfactory progress." Do these procedures seem to conform to acceptable standards of "reasonableness"?

THE JUDICIAL SYSTEM

Cases come before the judicial system in order to resolve legal controversies. In these controversies, lawyers present evidence to determine facts. It is not always simple to determine the facts when human nature is involved; different people have different interpretations of events. When the facts are incontrovertible, the question to be determined is typically one of application or interpretation of the law. Such cases are determined by a judge or magistrate rather than a jury.

Jurisdiction

Courts can only take cases under their jurisdiction. Each court has the authority to hear certain cases. The judicial process is also tiered into two basic sections: state and federal. Although the system varies from state to state, there are typically three sub tiers to state court systems. The first level is the trial court, followed by the intermediate court of appeals, and the final court of appeals. The federal system also consists of three tiers: original trial court, intermediate federal court of appeals, and finally the U.S. Supreme Court. A case may be appealed from a lower court to a higher court to be heard again. Such appeals are not always granted.

TRIAL PROCESS

Some cases are settled out of court while others go to trial. A trial always involves a plaintiff and a defendant. This two-party method of trying cases is known as an adversarial proceeding. In pleading and pretrial motions, documents that set forth the facts as perceived by plaintiff and defendant are developed. These serve as a basis for the legal claims of each party. The plaintiff and defendant question witnesses, seek depositions, and collect evidence to be used during the discovery, pretrial procurement, or trial.

The important process of discovery commences after suit is filed. The purpose of discovery is to obtain as much information as is possible from your opponent. This is done by way of interrogatories (written questions), requests for production of documents, depositions, and requests for admission of facts, among others.

Pretrial motions are a form of pleadings. Pleadings are any written documents filed by a party in a lawsuit. Frequently, pretrial motions will deal with discovery issues such as an opponent's failure to produce documents or when, where, and what type of deposition can be taken.

The actual trial is the legal proceeding during which evidence is collected, facts are determined, principles of law are applied, and a solution or verdict is reached. This judgment is made by the presiding judge when the appeals process is complete. Figure 9–1 shows the steps in a typical suit.

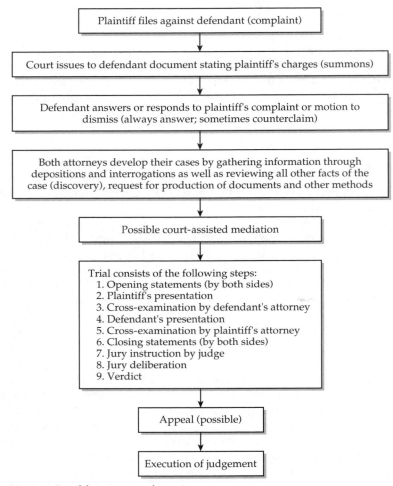

FIGURE 9–1. Possible steps in a lawsuit.

Statute of Limitations

Time limits exist for the filing of most suits or criminal charges. These are known as statutes of limitations. In Alabama, not all charges have a statute of limitations (for example, the crime of rape does not). In the case of an automobile accident, the injured party has 2 years to bring a cause of action against the one causing damages. If he or she fails to do so, the case will be lost procedurally regardless of merit. Traumatic injury cases have strict statutes of limitation because the injured party should be immediately aware of the injury. It is wise to file as soon as possible anyway, as it becomes increasingly difficult to gather accurate evidence with the passage of time.

The statute of limitations differs for minors because of the "disability" of minority. The law permits a minor's claim to be extended from the time of majority (typically age 18 or 19) plus the time specified in the statute for the particular cause of action. Law can typically be categorized as criminal or civil. The following is a discussion of both; however, most cases in health care involve civil liability.

CRIMINAL LIABILITY

Criminal law is all federal, state, or local law that broadly deals with crime and its punishment; crimes are subdivided into felonies and misdemeanors. Criminal law, like all law, is enacted to prevent harm to society. Substantive criminal laws are commonly codified into criminal or penal codes governing arrest, search, seizure, bail, and so on.

Two elements must exist for an individual to be convicted of a crime: a criminal act (*actus reas*) and criminal intent (*mens reas*). Thus, a jury may rule an act not criminal if the act was involuntary or accidental, if the person could not understand that the act was criminal, or if the act was necessary, as in self-defense. Once an individual has been tried on a criminal charge, he or she cannot be tried again for the same charge. This is the U.S. Constitutional bar against double jeopardy (Fifth Amendment).

There are a number of forms of punishment for crimes: monetary fines, removal of privileges (such as state licenses), parole, imprisonment, or, in the most extreme cases, execution.

Crimes that could possibly involve a health-care professional such as a medical imaging professional during practice include criminal violations associated with licensure or safe practice (e.g., medication administration outside the scope of practice or state licensure) and society's pandemic, drug abuse (covered in Chap. 6).

Felonies

Felonies are serious criminal offenses that are typically punished by severe penalties such as incarceration in excess of 1 year or fines in excess of $1000. Murder, manslaughter, kidnapping, and controlled substance violations (trafficking) are typical felonies.

Although it is a rare and unconscionable occurrence, health-care professionals are occasionally accused of murder or manslaughter within the execution of their duties. Such cases typically involve nurses or other professionals who inject a patient with lethal substances. Charges of kidnapping have been brought against health-care professionals who have had individuals committed to mental institutions against their will and without sound reason.

A felony conviction often results in a health-care professional being unable to become certified or licensed by a state or national certifying body.

A health-care professional who is already certified or licensed could lose certification or licensure, sometimes permanently.

Misdemeanors

A felony charge against a health-care professional during practice is extremely rare; misdemeanors are more common. A misdemeanor is loosely defined as any crime that is not a felony. Some related to health care include criminally negligent manslaughter, failure to report certain injuries or illnesses, failure to provide emergency services, fraudulent business activities, and violations of professional practice acts or health and safety codes.

CIVIL LIABILITY

Civil law is any law that is noncriminal. In civil lawsuits, the individual filing the suit is the plaintiff or petitioner, and the individual or group against which the claim is made is the defendant or respondent.

Most civil suits are punishable by damages in the form of monetary compensation decided on by the judge or jury. Whereas in criminal cases, the burden of proof must be beyond a reasonable doubt, in civil cases the burden of proof is by a preponderance of evidence. There are many types of civil law, including contract, labor, patent, and (the most common for individual claims against health-care workers) tort law.

A tort is a wrongful act (outside of breach of contract) committed against a person or property. Tort law exists to preserve peace among individuals by providing a substitute for vengeance, to find fault for wrongdoing (culpability), to deter the wrongdoer, and to provide compensation for injured persons.

Unintentional Torts

Acts that are not intended to do harm but still result in damage to person or property are unintentional torts. Negligence and malpractice are usually unintentional torts. Failing to provide for a patient's safety, carry out orders, or properly educate the patient (e.g., proper follow-up instructions were not given after a diagnostic procedure and the patient was injured or damaged in some way) are some examples of actions that could lead to a charge of malpractice against a medical imaging professional.

Malpractice and negligence will be covered in greater detail in Chapter 10, with special focus on preventing malpractice claims.

Intentional Torts

An intentional tort requires willful action. Three elements are necessary to consider a tort intentional: (1) the defendant's act was intended to interfere with the plaintiff or property belonging to the plaintiff; (2) the consequences of the act were also intended; and (3) the act was a substantial factor in bringing about the consequences.

Assault

An assault is an act that causes another person to fear that he or she will be touched in an offensive, insulting, or physically injurious manner without consent or authority to do so. An assault can be a raising of the fist or a threat to a noncompliant patient, in which the victim was in reasonable apprehension of immediate bodily harm.

Battery

Assault is typically coupled with battery. Battery is the actual act of harmful or unwarranted or unconsented contact with a person. Simple touching without permission is battery. Unwarranted performance of a medical imaging procedure might also be considered battery.

False Imprisonment

False imprisonment is the illegal detention of a person without consent. It may be making a patient stay in an area by not allowing him or her to leave, or as discussed in Chapter 10 the use of restraints. False imprisonment requires: (1) confinement of a victim, (2) intent to do so by the perpetrator, and (3) lack of consent by the victim. Giving a patient medication that does not allow him or her to leave the facility might also be considered false imprisonment, and can lead to other charges.

Intentional Infliction of Emotional Distress

This is also known as the tort of outrage and may be associated with the above three torts. Making disparaging remarks concerning a patient or making fun of his or her problem might cause the patient emotional distress. These actions go so far beyond the courtesy and care expected of a health-care worker that they are, indeed, outrageous. This tort requires that: (1) the perpetrator knew or should have known that the conduct would cause emotional distress; (2) the conduct was extreme and outrageous; (3) the perpetrator's actions were the cause of distress; and (4) the distress was severe and no reasonable person should have to endure it.

A relevant case is *Johnson v Woman's Hospital*.[9] The plaintiff's child was stillborn, and she was given assurance that the child would be buried in what she considered to be an acceptable manner. Following a reading of the pathologist's report, however, it appeared that the baby was not buried in the manner she believed.

Returning to the hospital, Mrs. Johnson asked about the disposition of her infant's body. A nurse employed by the hospital simply handed her a gallon container with the shriveled body of the infant floating in formaldehyde. The conduct of the hospital and nurse was found to be outrageous, and the Johnsons were awarded $100,000 for the emotional distress inflicted upon them.

Another case was *McCormick v Haley*,[10] in which a physician's office sent a reminder letter to a patient to come in for a checkup, even though the patient had died. Two additional reminder letters came after a suit was filed by the decedent's husband; the court ruled that the first letter could be considered a mistake, but the second and third could be the basis for liability.

Quasi-Intentional Torts

In quasi-intentional torts, there may not have been an intent to injure or distress a patient, but the act was voluntary and did result in injury or distress. These torts, in the health-care setting, violate personal reputation or privacy.

Defamation of Character

Defamation of character is the invasion of a person's reputation and good name, and includes slander and libel. Slander is a false oral statement that damages a person's reputation, whereas libel is a false written or representational statement that damages a reputation. False statements about people, whether spoken or written, can be very damaging. Consider the following: A 17-year-old girl was admitted through the emergency room with acute abdominal pain. She was transported to the radiology department by an attendant for abdominal films. The attendant noticed on the patient's chart the initials PID. The attendant thought that the patient had a venereal disease. When the patient asked the attendant if he knew what was wrong with her, he told her she had syphilis.

After leaving her in radiology for her procedure, the attendant dropped off a note to a friend in central supply giving the name and illness of the patient. The young man in central supply was a high school classmate of the patient.

When the patient returned to the emergency room, she told her family that the attendant said she had syphilis. They immediately demanded that the physician explain their daughter's condition to them. The physician assured the family that the young woman did not have syphilis, but rather pelvic inflammatory disease. The doctor apologized for the attendant's behavior. After the patient was released from the hospital, her family filed suit against the hospital for defamation of character.

In this case, there are several possible liabilities. First, the attendant verbally slandered the patient when he said she had syphilis (which she did not). Second, he committed libel because he wrote this information down for his friend in central supply to read. The young woman could claim that her reputation was damaged, particularly since the worker in central supply was her high school classmate. The patient's privacy was also invaded since her medical records were disclosed without consent.[11]

Invasion of Privacy

Invasion of privacy is a violation of a person's right to protection against unreasonable and unwarranted interference. A seminal case establishing the patient's right to privacy was *Inderbitzem v Lane Hospital*, in which rectal and vaginal examinations were performed repeatedly on a patient by medical students, even though she requested that they not do so.[12]

One type of invasion of privacy is breech of confidentiality, in which a person's trust and confidence are violated by public revelation of confidential or privileged information without that person's consent. If a patient's picture were inappropriately published in a local newspaper, this would be an invasion of privacy. The Code of Federal Regulations prohibits the release of information concerning patients being treated for substance abuse or related conditions.[13] For radiographic film evaluation sessions, instructors in radiography and other diagnostic imaging programs typically encourage students to cut off or otherwise block off the names of patients to prevent potential invasion of privacy.

Another potential invasion of privacy of particular importance to medical imaging professionals is improper covering of a patient, or the unnecessary exposure of portions of the patient's body during the course of a procedure. It is very important that the patient be kept covered. Any unnecessary exposure of portions of a patient's body, especially the genitals, could result in charges of invasion of privacy.

LEGAL DOCTRINES

To better understand torts, one must also consider a number of doctrines relevant to the practice of medical imaging and other health-care professionals.

Respondeat Superior

The legal doctrine *respondeat superior* ("let the master answer") states that an employer will be held liable for an employee's negligent act. Independent contractors are typically responsible for their own acts. Two conditions must typically exist for this doctrine to be applicable: (1) an employer-employee relationship must exist and (2) the employee must be functioning under the authority of the employer. Principal-agent relationships are also subject to *respondeat superior.* The master-servant relationship exists whenever the employer has a right to control the employee's activities, supervise the employee in the performance of job-related tasks, pay a wage, and discharge the employee at any time.[14,15]

A supervisor is not an employer under *respondeat superior,* but a supervisor can be held responsible for personal acts or omissions, as well as be liable for improper supervision or improper provision of care.[16]

Doctrine of Corporate Responsibility

Although early hospitals may have viewed themselves similar to hotels that rented space and resources to physicians and patients, this view has not been found acceptable.[17] Decisions in the 1950s and 1960s found the hospital liable to fulfill directly duties to the patients. These included procedures to count sponges[18] and the taking of patient histories in the radiology department.[19]

Although the application of corporate responsibility seems to vary from state to state,[20] the classic case *Darling v Charleston Community Memorial Hospital* seems to reflect the predominant view of the hospital's liability.[21] Mr. Darling was a football player and had a constrictive case applied that caused circulatory complications that led to gangrene. These complications were not communicated by the nursing staff to the medical staff. The patient's leg had to be amputated. The Illinois Supreme Court found that the hospital could be held accountable for the actions of its staff.

Doctrine of Borrowed Servant

This is often considered in tandem with *respondeat superior.* Employees may be "borrowed" for a specific purpose. The law infers that the one controlling or directing the employee has greater responsibility than the one paying the employee.

A relevant case is the radiographer assisting a radiologist with a procedure. Radiologists are often independent contractors, whereas radiographers are typically employed by the institution. The radiologist has control over the radiographer when performing procedures and thus may be seen to have the greater liability. This doctrine does not, however, rule out liability on the part of the hospital or radiographer.

Captain of the Ship

A person in charge (captain) may be held responsible for all of those under his or her supervision (crew). For example, in surgery, a team is often assembled consisting of a surgeon, a nurse-anesthetist, surgical nurses, and perhaps a surgeon's assistant and a radiographer. The surgeon may be seen as the team leader (or "captain of the ship"), and thus takes ultimate responsibility for the actions of the team members. Again, this does not necessarily remove responsibility from other members of the team for their own actions. This principle is, for the most part, outmoded and not followed in most jurisdictions today due to more medically related lawsuits being specific to the person or persons thought responsible.

Doctrine of Personal Liability

This is a fundamental rule of law that holds each person responsible for his or her own tortious conduct, even though others may be liable as well. This rule should be remembered in situations in which an authority figure such as a physician assures the medical imaging professional that he or she will take responsibility for an action. As a professional, the medical imager is responsible for his or her own actions (or lack of action) and cannot use as a defense, the statement that "The doctor said it was OK."

Doctrine of the Reasonably Prudent Man

This doctrine is applicable to the patient as well as to the health-care professional. Individuals performing an action are expected to perform that action as would any reasonable person of ordinary prudence. Health-care professionals are expected to perform prudently as would those of similar education, training, and skills.

The reasonably prudent man standard is often applied in situations of patient consent. For example, a patient who may not have been informed of the risk of death, may die from injection of contrast media. In such a case, the jury must decide if the remote risk of death would have discouraged the patient, as a reasonably prudent person, from undergoing the examination.

Res Ipsa Loquitur

The doctrine of *res ipsa loquitur* ("the act or thing speaks for itself") holds that the cause of the negligence is obvious. In such cases no legal expert testimony may be needed. However, in most cases, the word of a medical expert is needed to establish the fact that an act was negligent.

One of the classic examples of negligence involving *res ipsa* is leaving sponges or instruments in a patient following surgery. However, the conditions of *res ipsa* are not absolute; for example, if an emergency required that the patient be sutured immediately, and there was no time for a sponge count, the surgeon would not be viewed as acting negligently.

CONCLUSION

This chapter has provided the student of medical imaging with a basic introduction to the concepts of law as well as relevant definitions. Although some examples were provided, Chapter 10 gives more specific examples in the application of law to the practice of medical imaging.

REFERENCES

1. LeGrys, VA, Beck, SJ, and Laudicina, RJ: Legal aspects associated with dismissal from clinical laboratory science programs. Clinical Laboratory Science 8:219–225, 1995.
2. Roe v Wade (410 US 113).
3. Dowd, SB, and Proud, K: Wrongful birth and ultrasonography: Legal and ethical issues. Today's Ethics Journal 1:1–19, 1994.
4. Smith v Cote 513 A2d 341 (NH 1986).
5. Proffitt v Bartolo 412 NW 2d 232 (Mich Ct App 1987).
6. Ward, MD, and Diaz, A: What radiologic technology educators should know about due process of law. Radiol Technol 60:3, 1989.
7. Horowitz v Board of Curators of the University of Missouri, 435 US 78 (1978).
8. Regents of University of Michigan v Ewing, 474 US 214 (1985).
9. Johnson v Woman's Hospital, 527 SW 133 (Tenn Ct App 1975).
10. McCormick v Haley, 307 NE 2d 34 (Ohio App 1973).
11. Parelli, RJ: Medicolegal Issues for Radiographers. Dubuque, IA, Shepherd, 1991, pp 4–6, Vignette 2.
12. Inderbitzen v Lane Hospital, 124 Cal App 462, 12 P 2d 744 (1932).
13. 42 CFR Part 2.
14. State Department of Industrial Relations v Montgomery Baptist Hospital, 359 S 2d 410 (Al Civ App 1978).
15. Code of Alabama, 1975, Section 25-4-8.
16. Miller, RD: Liability and the supervisor. Health Care Supervisor 1(2):59–72, 1983.
17. Annas, G: The Rights of Patients, ed 2. Carbondale, Ill, Southern Illinois Press, 1989.
18. Leonard v Watsonville Community Hospital, 47 Cal 2d 509, 305 P 2d 36 (1957).
19. Favalora v Aetna Casualty & Surety Co, 144 So 2d 544 (La Ct App 1962).
20. Ruse, RE: Introduction to health law. Seminars in Radiologic Technology 2:112–120, 1994.
21. Darling v Charleston Community Memorial Hospital, 211 NE2d 253 (1965).

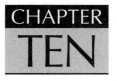

CHAPTER TEN

Medical Legal Issues for the Practice of Medical Imaging

Sharon B. Barnes, MPH, ARRT(R)
Steven B. Dowd, EdD, ARRT(R)
Jane Faulkner Evans, JD, ARRT(R)(NMT)

This chapter discusses some of the medical legal issues relevant to the clinical practice of medical imaging professionals. Standard of care and scope of practice will be covered, especially as each relates to preventing malpractice. Five issues with legal implications will then be discussed: confidentiality and medical records, death and dying, communicable diseases, false imprisonment, and the proper use of radiographic equipment and ionizing radiation.

OBJECTIVES

At the end of this chapter, the reader will be able to:

- Discuss Standard of Care and Scope of Practice
- Define malpractice
- Discuss the incidence of malpractice in radiology
- List means through which the medical imaging professional can prevent malpractice
- Describe the liability for disclosure of confidential information
- Discuss the legal means by which society has addressed the ethical problems of euthanasia and death and dying
- Discuss the legal obligations of employees in treating patients with communicable diseases

- List some relevant organizations that develop and implement regulations for the proper use of ionizing radiation
- Discuss law relevant to the safe operation of equipment
- List reasons why radiation exposure lawsuits are uncommon and difficult for the plaintiff

STANDARD OF CARE

Professionals owe a certain degree or standard of care to the patient. In the State of Alabama, for example, the following standards have been set for physicians, dentists, and surgeons.

1. In performing professional services for a patient, a physician's, surgeon's, or dentist's duty to the patient shall be to exercise such reasonable care, diligence and skill as physicians, surgeons, and dentists in the same general neighborhood, and in the same general line of practice, ordinarily have and exercise in a like case. In the case of a hospital rendering services to a patient, the hospital must use that degree of care, skill, and diligence used by hospitals generally in the community.
2. Neither a physician, surgeon, dentist, nor hospital shall be considered an insurer of the successful issue of treatment or service.[1]

According to a ruling in *Lamont v Brookwood Health Services, Inc,*[2] the phrase "that degree of care, skill, and diligence used by hospitals generally in the community" refers to the national hospital community. *Thomasson v Dicthelm*[3] clarified the role of legislation in addressing liability of medical professionals in the context of patient-doctor and patient-hospital relationships.

Duties of Medical Imaging Professionals

Just as physicians must provide a standard of care, medical imaging professionals are also expected to provide a certain standard of care, which is applied in medical malpractice cases. Lack of education or experience is not an acceptable excuse for a lack of care. For example, a radiographer who is working as a radiation therapist without having attended a radiation therapy program or passed the credentialing examination will be held to the same standards as practicing radiation therapists with education and credentials in that discipline.

One way of ensuring that appropriately current standards of care are being practiced is through continuing education and other means of maintaining currency, such as reading journal articles. Attorneys defending a medical imaging professional in a malpractice suit use *Radiologic Technology* or other professional journals to determine if appropriate and current standards of care were followed. Appropriate standards of care could also be established through textbooks for imaging professionals and hospital procedure manuals or through radiology department policy and procedure manuals.

SCOPE OF PRACTICE

The Scope of Practice, as developed by the American Society of Radiologic Technologists (ASRT) and other professional organizations, is one of many documents that defines the working life of a medical imaging professional and the expected standard of care. Other important documents include the job description, licensure laws, and codes of ethics.

The following case described by Skotnik[4] is an example of malpractice for operating outside the scope of practice. Technologists at a freestanding imaging center administered an unspecified amount of chloral hydrate to sedate a child. The concentration, amount, and type of drug were not documented. The child was unconscious when taken home, where she died the same day from acute chloral hydrate poisoning.

The technologists and the radiologist were found liable as part of a 34.65-million-dollar lawsuit on the grounds that there was a clear violation in the Scope of Practice: Technologists may not, other than as a part of contrast administration, administer drugs to a patient. The scope of practice, however, is not static. The need for multiskilled professionals may force expansion of the scope of practice. This is evidenced by the inclusion of pharmacology in radiologic science professional curricula.

In 1991, the ASRT added venipuncture to the scope of practice for radiographers (venipuncture has always been considered an integral component of the work of nuclear medicine technologists). In a survey of state regulations, Tortorici and MacDonald[5] found that California and New York specifically prohibit radiographers from performing venipuncture and that New Jersey specifically forbids both venipuncture and the injection of contrast or other drugs by radiographers. Obviously, in these states, radiographers cannot perform venipuncture even though the ASRT Scope of Practice includes this task. In some states, venipuncture is included in relevant regulations such as licensure laws (Illinois, Montana, and Utah are examples); in others, it is not so clear.

> **DISCUSSION QUESTION**
> List the positive and negative aspects of licensure, Scope of Practice, and job descriptions. What value does each serve to the worker? To the patient? How can these documents be made more valuable?

MALPRACTICE

Malpractice is the failure to do something that a reasonable person, guided by those considerations which ordinarily regulate human affairs, would do, or the doing of something that a reasonable person would not do.[6] Negligence, a similar term and the parent of malpractice, is a breach or failure to fulfill the expected standard of care. Duty, breach of duty, injury, and proximate cause of an injury must all be shown. Although it is not a common occurrence, medical imaging professionals can be and have been sued for malpractice.

Medical malpractice cases, according to one report, have increased 100% in the last 10 years.[7] Eleven of every one hundred dollars paid by patients to physicians goes to malpractice insurance.[8] Only 1 of every 10 patients whose injury is due to negligence files a claim.[9] Indeed, several attorneys consulted by the authors suggest that cases of medical malpractice are decreasing. Since medical malpractice is a complex issue, caution should be used when interpreting the results of empirical studies on the subject.[10] Malpractice claim rates and awards vary from state to state, and by the time the results of a study are published, the data analyzed may be outdated.

DISCUSSION QUESTION

Ralph is an MRI technologist working in a facility that allows him to administer a variety of medications to patients. He has not received any special training in the use of medications except undocumented on-the-job training. Although his facility has assured him that they will stand behind him, only physicians and nurses in his state may inject.

One day, Ralph's patient has a cardiac arrest when he administers a sedative. The patient recovers, but must spend 5 extra days in the hospital. What is the likely outcome if a malpractice case is pursued surrounding the administration of medication by Ralph?

Civil Suits for Medical Malpractice

Lawsuits are structured and conducted according to state or federal rules of civil/criminal procedure. This was described in some detail in Chapter 9. The courts have two main concerns: (1) to resolve the dispute between the parties according to the rules of law and (2) to accomplish this resolution within a fixed time period as required by state law.

Attorneys must follow the rules of civil practice and procedure and ascertain that there are valid grounds for a lawsuit. Both a party to a suit and the attorney can be sanctioned for filing a frivolous lawsuit.

It is very important for an attorney, on the first interview with the client, to ascertain the facts, the causes, the injury, the date or discovery of the injury, and whether it is reasonable that the defendant caused such injury or damages to the plaintiff.

Out-of-Court Settlements

According to Skotnik,[4] most disputes do not lead to lawsuits but rather to out-of-court settlements. Since many cases are settled before going to trial, it is difficult to determine what really happened. This provides little guidance for the technologist wanting to know proper action. But if the majority of lawsuits were not settled before trial, the U.S. Courts could become so overwhelmed that judicial gridlock might occur.

Malpractice in Radiology

A survey by Hollingsworth[11] found that, of 415 radiology-related lawsuits 88% were related to staff, with 24% of these involving improperly performed procedures and 11% involving patient falls. Radiographers appear to be called to court most often in cases of patient falls.

About 12% of all medical malpractice cases involve radiologists.[12] These cases are approximately evenly divided between "failure to diagnose" and procedural suits. Failure to diagnose typically involves missed fractures or failure to diagnose cancer. Procedural suits typically involve complications. However, one study found that disputes over informed consent were common in radiology, with 8% of radiologists surveyed reporting involvement in informed consent litigation.[13]

A study by Barloon and Shumway[14] of radiologic colon examinations found that about 50% of cases were brought on behalf of decedents. Plaintiffs charged that a failure to diagnose colorectal cancer led to a delay in treatment that caused a patient's death. The other cases primarily involved perforation of the colon. Gelfand[15] made the following interesting comment about the study:

> Only well-trained technologists [should be] employed to staff the fluoro-scopic suite. This practice would ensure that an experienced person would insert the enema tip and would increase the likelihood that the barium examination will be of satisfactory technical quality. An inexperienced technologist or a student technologist should never be allowed to insert an enema tip without supervision.

An interesting survey of medical malpractice in pediatric medical imaging that is relevant to general medical imaging is summarized in Box 10–1.[16]

Box 10–1. MALPRACTICE IN PEDIATRIC RADIOLOGY

Sample: Chairs of pediatric radiology departments in pediatric hospitals
Malpractice premiums paid per radiologist per year: $499–$29,000 (mean = $8,630)
Largest number of claims: Gastrointestinal/abdominal and thoracic radiography (This may indicate a lack of attention to "routine" practice, since these were also identified as "less risky.")
Length of cases: 0–12 years (mean = 3.9 years)
Number of cases going to trial: 1 (of 28)
Settlements: $500,000–$1,500,000 (1 case); $500,000 (1 case); $25,000–$175,000 (4 cases); less than $25,000 (4 cases)
Areas seen as higher risk: Interventional procedures, angiography, sedation, neuroradiology
Areas seen as lower risk: Gastrointestinal procedure, teleradiology, genetics, chest, and fax confidentiality

---

The Medical Imaging Professional's Role in Preventing Malpractice Suits

Medical imaging professionals can prevent malpractice suits through commonsense adherence to principles of good practice and by maintaining currency in skills and knowledge. Additionally, adherence to the "7 Cs" listed in Box 10–2 can help as well. Remember that medical imaging professionals are, first and foremost, patient advocates, and second, assistants to physicians.

Many practitioners complain that malpractice cases are retrospective in nature; that is, they start from an adverse event and work their way back to determine what the professional "should have done." In many malpractice cases, however, what should have been done is based on sound practice already known to the practitioner. For example, one malpractice claim in the Barloon and Shumway study involved overelevation of a barium bag—something every radiographer knows to be inappropriate.

CONFIDENTIALITY

The fear of litigation makes the custodian of medical records cautious. The release of confidential information is based on (1) the authorization of the patient; (2) a judicial mandate by issuance of a subpoena duces tecum; and (3) a statutory mandate, such as those for reporting communicable disease or child abuse. All states have laws regarding the proper maintenance of medical records. The average length of maintenance of radiographs is 5 years, except in the case of minors, where it is usually to the age of consent plus a time period of 1 to 7 years.[17]

Medical images are part of a patient's medical records, which are typi-

---

Box 10–2. THE 7 Cs OF MALPRACTICE PREVENTION

1. **Competence.** Maintain certification, participate in continuing education, and follow the current literature.
2. **Compliance.** Follow policies and procedures established for the radiology department. Policies and procedures should be reread on a yearly basis.
3. **Charting.** The chart is a legal document; the two most important aspects of charting are accuracy and timeliness.
4. **Communications.** Verbal and nonverbal communication skills are equally important. This includes a clean x-ray room, neat personal appearance, and courteous manner in dealing with the patients, patient's family members, and other members of the hospital staff. Some estimate that 90% of lawsuits could be eliminated through proper communication.
5. **Confidentiality.** Ensure that no information on a patient is released to anyone not entitled to know without a properly signed release, medical authorization, or a court subpoena.
6. **Courtesy.** Be courteous in dealing with patients, patient's family members, and other members of the hospital staff, and treat all patients with equal dignity and respect.
7. **Carefulness.** Follow the basic guidelines for good practice that you learned in your professional education. They serve as a baseline, but also stay current in clinical practice.

Adapted from Tilke, B: Word to wise: It only takes one lawsuit. ADVANCE for Radiologic Technologists 3(34):6, 1990; and Dowd, SB: Medical Law and Ethics. Birmingham, Ala, University of Alabama at Birmingham, 1995.

---

cally owned by the hospital. They are never to be released without proper authorization, such as a subpoena duces tecum or a patient's release in writing.

Liability for Unauthorized Disclosure of Confidential Information

The willful revelation of information about a patient without proper authorization is a breach of confidentiality. In the case of *Hammonds v AETNA Casualty & Surety Company*,[18] an insurance company induced a physician to reveal confidential medical information to them. The court ruled for the plaintiff, saying that there was a legal and ethical duty to keep patient information confidential. The physician breached his duty of protection and disclosed confidential information. The court ruled that anyone who induces a physician to divulge confidential information in violation of the physician's legal responsibility to the patient may be held liable in damages to the patient under Ohio law.

In a 1973 Alabama case, *Horne v Patton*,[19] a physician revealed medical data to a patient's employer without authorization, resulting in the termination of the job of the patient/employee. The court held that an employer does not necessarily have a legitimate interest in an employee's health history.

Legal Obligation to Disclose

There is a misconception among many health-care professionals that the *ethical* practice of maintaining confidentiality will provide *legal* protection for failure to disclose information as required by law or to protect society. However, just as newspaper reporters can be sent to jail for not revealing confidential sources, health-care professionals can be held liable for not revealing confidential information when legally requested.

The best-known example in health care is the 1974 Tarasoff decision, which held that psychotherapists must warn potential victims of violence.[20] This case was reheard in 1976, and the new ruling emphasized professional judgment on the part of the therapist, broadening the therapist's responsibility to protect and not simply warn. The ruling placed responsibility on the physician to warn or protect society from potential harm. In other words, the obligation to society was greater than the obligation to the patient with regard to confidentiality. This ruling has implications for a variety of practice settings, including the treatment of children and families, sexual misconduct by health-care professionals, HIV-positive patients, and assessment of patient's abilities.

Simply put, health-care professionals, including medical imaging professionals, must understand both the law and the ethical demands of their profession and patient care to know when to reveal information and when information should be withheld.

> **DISCUSSION QUESTION**
> One issue that often arises in the medical imaging department is the patient who wants to read his or her chart. The technologist must hold this information confidential because the patient's attending physician is normally the person who relates diagnostic information to the patient. Discuss the best way to handle such patients.

EUTHANASIA

Many practitioners will face decisions regarding a patient's rights. The American Hospital Association has published a Bill of Rights for patients. Patients also have other rights, including the right to decide how to die.

The first precept of this right is that the patient has the right to be treated as a living human being until he or she dies.[21] Stark in its simplicity and logic, this precept is not universally followed. What complicates our view of death is that most Americans do not support active euthanasia as practiced by Dr. Kervorkian. Active euthanasia, or the act of hastening death, is seen as morally suspect because it is difficult to determine when a patient is actually "terminal."

Although most Americans do support passive euthanasia, which allows the dying individual to choose his or her environment and treatment while dying, it is often difficult to distinguish between the two. For that reason, for many years society tended to shun the dying; it was easier to simply ignore the problem.

Recently, society has addressed this problem through legal means with the Patient Self-Determination Act.[22] Health-care providers and institutions that receive Medicare or Medicaid funding must inform patients of their legal rights to accept or refuse medical or surgical treatment, as well as the right to formulate advanced directives. Advanced directives are documents, such as a living will or durable power of attorney for health care, that relate to the provision of health care once the individual is incapacitated. Although Americans may not be willing to let individuals hasten or bring about their own death, our laws have changed in recent years to allow individuals to die when they are terminally ill.

DISCUSSION QUESTION

A patient with an advanced directive that includes a DNR (do not resuscitate) order is undergoing an angiogram. You are the lead technologist. The patient experiences cardiac arrest, and the radiologist begins the resuscitation process. When you remind him of the DNR, he brushes you aside and instructs you to assist him in the resuscitation process. What do you do? Include in your discussion legal and ethical concerns such as state law, *Respondeat Superior* (see Chap. 9), patient autonomy, and the role of the medical imaging professional as patient advocate and physician assistant. Consider the following as well: What would the legal penalty be for saving a patient's life? Also note that once heroic measures have begun, in most cases they cannot be terminated.

TREATMENT OF PATIENTS WITH COMMUNICABLE OR CONTAGIOUS DISEASES

In Chapter 7, we noted that medical imaging professionals are ethically obligated to treat patients with communicable diseases such as AIDS. However, a health-care worker may be basing refusal to treat such patients on an institution's failure to provide proper infection control practices. This action may be protected under the Occupational Safety and Health Act (OSHA).[23] OSHA allows employees to refuse to work, and forbids their discharge, if, in good faith, they believe that the workplace poses an immediate and grave danger to their health and safety.

The hospital or facility is responsible for determining the reason for an employee's refusal to work with certain groups of patients. In some cases, reasonable accommodation must be made if the employee has a valid medical reason for refusal. If a hospital is following proper infection control procedures and properly educates the employee regarding the transmittal of the HIV virus, for example, then the hospital can institute disciplinary action, including terminating the employee.[24]

DISCUSSION QUESTION

Discuss reasonable accommodations for employees who do not want to work with patients with a communicable disease. Also discuss what arguments you would use to convince someone who is otherwise able but unwilling to treat such patients.

FALSE IMPRISONMENT

Patients may bring about a charge of false imprisonment if they feel they have been confined against their will. This may include general considerations, such as not being allowed to make a telephone call, or more specific to imaging, the use of patient restraints.

Some medical imaging professionals may use restraints to secure certain projections on patients (and many patients in long-term care facilities are already restrained) and should be aware of problems that can result. The problem is not so acute with children or individuals who have been deemed "incompetent," but it may be with elderly patients who are frail and need assistance but may misinterpret the use of restraints. Many state elder abuse statutes include "unreasonable confinement" as a means of abuse, and the restraints used in imaging may be seen as a form of unreasonable confinement if consent is not secured or the restraints are not used in accordance with departmental policy and procedure. Although governmental regulations such as the Omnibus Reconciliation Act (OBRA) of 1987 increasingly mitigate against the use of restraints, health-care facilities still tend to overuse restraints.[25,26]

A health-care facility can lose its funding for misusing restraints. Robbins and associates[27] also found that restrained hospital patients were eight times more likely to die than those who were not. Despite these drawbacks and the loss of patient dignity and possible charges of elder abuse, a study by Janelli and associates[28] found that over 64% of nursing home staff members felt a legal obligation (e.g., fear of being sued) to use restraints for patient safety.

RADIATION PROTECTION LAWS

Most radiation protection laws are enacted at the state level because the U.S. Constitution invests the promotion of citizen's health in the states.[29] There are a number of federal guidelines as well, especially in nuclear medicine, which is much more heavily regulated than the practice of radiology. Of course, this situation can change; if regulations similar to the Mammography Quality Standards Act (MQSA) are implemented in general radiology or if a national health-care bill ever passes, radiology may also be strongly regulated at the federal level.

THE FORMATION OF REGULATIONS

The organizations that promulgate regulations in medical imaging are the U.S. Nuclear Regulatory Commission (NRC), the Food and Drug Administration (FDA), and the Environmental Protection Agency (EPA). There are also various regulations related to Medicare and state requirements. Recommendations from the Conference of Radiation Control Program Directors (CRCPD) and other organizations may be the source of many of these regulations.

For example, the FDA regulates the design and manufacture of electronic products such as x-ray equipment. It spot-checks equipment installed in the United States to check compliance with items such as beam quality, linearity of mA stations, and collimation. The FDA also initiated a Safe Medical Devices Act,[30] which requires professionals such as radiographers to report defects in equipment that "has caused or contributed to the death of a patient or a serious injury or serious illness of a patient." This act carries fines for failure to report.

The rights of patients to reasonably adequate equipment was established some years ago in the case of *Arterburn v St. Joseph Hospital and Rehabilitation Center*.[31] This does not mean, however, that only the most up-to-date equipment is allowed; the case of *Lauro v. Travelers Insurance Co.*[32] showed that reasonably functioning older equipment is acceptable even when newer and more accurate equipment is available.

Radiation Exposure Lawsuits

In the early days of radiology (turn of the century), there were many lawsuits related to the improper use of x radiation, causing severe erythema, or Roentgen-ray burns. In severe cases, digits and limbs had to be amputated.[33]

With today's scientific use of x ray and other forms of radiation, such suits are no longer seen.

Legally, radiation exposure cases should be seen in the same light as environmental cases (e.g., toxic chemicals). There are many problems, though, for a patient or individual who wants to prove harm from low levels of ionizing radiation.[34] The largest problem is proving causation. It is difficult to say, for example, that radiation was the agent responsible for causing a person's cancer—any cancer caused by radiation can come about through natural means as well. Statutes of limitation apply (many cancers due to radiation take 30 or 40 years to develop) and proximate cause must be shown. However, one also cannot predict what will happen in any one court case, especially juried cases.

The Pregnant Employee

Although there have been a number of court decisions regarding the pregnant worker's right to work, two have special impact on medical imaging professionals. The first, *Hayes v Shelby Memorial Hospital*, found that a hospital could not contend that a state of "nonpregnancy" was a bona fide reason for termination.[35] A Supreme Court decision (*International Union [UAW] v Johnson Controls*) found that reassignment or termination of *pregnant* employees from so-called hazardous areas was not appropriate.[36]

State and federal regulations dealing with the use of ionizing radiation call for pregnant workers to declare their pregnancy—making them a "declared pregnant woman"—so that employers can work with the employee in keeping radiation doses as low as possible during a pregnancy.

CONCLUSION

Medical imaging professionals need to understand the law, including the acceptable parameters of their practice, in order to avoid lawsuits directed at them and their employers. Again, refer to Box 10-2, the 7Cs of Malpractice Prevention. A professional also understands that the law merely sets acceptable standards of care, one that should be surpassed whenever possible. Professional credentialing agencies and societies, such as those whose codes of ethics and/or conduct are listed in Chapter 3; our personal values and work ethics; and, of course, our patients, demand our best. When we strive to do our best according to professional parameters, the likelihood of lawsuits should decrease significantly.

REFERENCES

1. Code of Alabama, 1975, 6-5-484.
2. Lamont v Brookwood Health Services, Inc, 446 So2d 1018 (ALA 1983).
3. Thomasson v Dicthelm, 457 So2d 397 (ALA 1984).

4. Skotnik, JH: Legal issues for radiologic technologists in clinical practice. Seminars in Radiologic Technology 2:129–136, 1994.
5. Tortorici, M, and MacDonald, J: RTs performing venipuncture: A survey of state regulations. Radiol Technol 64:368–372, 1993.
6. Black's Law Dictionary, ed 5. St Paul, Minn, West, 1979, p 930.
7. VanSonnenberg, E, Barton, JB, and Wittich, GR. Radiology and the law, with an emphasis on interventional radiology. Radiology 187:297–303, 1993.
8. Domenici, PV, and Koop, CE: Sue the doctor? There's a better way. The New York Times, June 6, 1991, A19, A25.
9. Danzon, PM: Medical Malpractice: Theory, Evidence, and Public Policy. Cambridge, Mass, Harvard University Press, 1985.
10. Taragin, MI, Martin, K, Shapiro, S, et al: Physician malpractice: Does the past predict the future? J Gen Intern Med 10:550–556, 1995.
11. Hollingsworth, DG: Liability issues for radiology managers. Radiology Management 12(2):40–50, 1990.
12. Berlin, L: Malpractice and radiologists. Update 1986: An 11.5 year perspective. Am J Roentgenol 147:1291–1298, 1986.
13. Bundy, AA: Radiology and the Law. Rockville, Md, Aspen, 1988.
14. Barloon, TJ, and Shumway, J: Medical malpractice involving radiologic colon examinations: A review of 38 recent cases. Am J Roentgenol 165:343–346, 1995.
15. Gelfand, DW: Medical malpractice involving barium enema examinations. Am J Roentgenol 165:347–348, 1995.
16. Royal, SA, Cloud, GA, and Atchison, WM. Malpractice in pediatric radiology: A survey in the United States and Canada. Pediatr Radiol 24:519–522, 1994.
17. Obergfell, AM: Law and Ethics in Diagnostic Imaging and Therapeutic Radiology. Philadelphia, WB Saunders, 1995.
18. Hammonds v AETNA Casualty & Surety Company, 243 F Supp 793 (OH 1965).
19. Horne v Patton 287 So2d 824 (ALA 1973).
20. Joseph, DI: Confidentiality versus the duty to protect: Foreseeable harm in the practice of psychiatry. JAMA 266:425, 1991.
21. Hayslip, B, and Panek, PE: Adult Development and Aging. New York, Harper and Row, 1989.
22. Patient Self-Determination Act. Pub L No 101-508, 104 Stat 291 (1990).
23. 29 USC §§ 102, 157.
24. Stepp v Review Board of Indiana Employment Security Division, 521 NE2d 350 (Ind Ct App 1988).
25. Health Care Financing Administration. Medicare/Medicaid Nursing Home Information: 1987–1988. Washington, DC, Government Printing Office, 1988.
26. Kapp, MB: Nursing home restraints and legal liability. J Leg Med 13:1–32, 1992.
27. Robbins, LE, Boyko, E, Lane, J, et al. Binding the elderly: A prospective study of the use of mechanical restraints in an acute care hospital. J Am Geriatr Soc 35:290–296, 1987.
28. Janelli, LM, Kanski, GW, Scherer, YK, et al. Physical restraints: Practice, attitudes, and knowledge among nursing staff. The Journal of Long-Term Care Administration, 1992 (Summer), pp 22–25.
29. Dowd, SB, and Archer, J: Radiation safety regulations: The evolution and development of standards. Radiology Management 16(1):39–45, 1994.
30. Pub L 101-629 (1990).
31. Arterburn v St Joseph Hosp & Rehabilitation Center, 551 P2d 886 (1976).
32. Lauro v Travelers Insurance Co, 261 So2d 261 (La App 1972) cert denied 262 So2d 787 (1972).
33. Dowd, SB: Practical Radiation Protection and Applied Radiobiology. Philadelphia, WB Saunders, 1994.
34. Pesto-Edwards, MM: Legal recourse for damages suffered from low-level radiation exposure. In Hendee, WR (ed): Health Effects of Low Level Radiation. Norwalk, Conn, Appleton-Century-Crofts, 1984, pp 181–192.
35. Hayes v Shelby Memorial Hospital, 726 F2d 1543 (11th Cir 1984).
36. International Union (UAW) v Johnson Controls, Inc, US Ct 1196 (1991).

CHAPTER ELEVEN

Administrative Ethics

Steven B. Dowd, EdD, ARRT(R)
Michael W. Drafke, MS, ARRT(R)

This chapter provides a diverse view of the role of ethics in the administration of imaging departments and services, with an emphasis on the role of the manager. A general overview of ethical pressures is provided and the tasks of a manager are discussed. The role of the manager as a moral agent with a number of responsibilities is the focus of the material.

OBJECTIVES

At the end of this chapter, the reader will be able to:
- Describe how ethics affect a manager
- Describe the role of the manager as a moral agent
- State the need for leadership in the imaging profession
- Relate ethical principles to the administration of imaging services
- Analyze ethical dilemmas relevant to imaging services

THE IMAGING MANAGER

Hospitals are complex places that require an optimum mix of workers and managers to succeed. The manager's four basic roles are planning, controlling, organizing, and directing, all of which make the organization more efficient. Managers must deal with human, financial, informational, and material resources. There are various types of managers in the hospital: the president or chief executive officer (CEO), division directors, department directors (e.g., director of the department of radiology), and a number of so-called middle managers who function as supervisors, or to use a more modern term, team leaders.

Imaging managers are typically professionals from an allied health area (radiography, nuclear medicine, or ultrasound) who have, through a combination of on-the-job experience and education, advanced into a management position. As professionals, they often feel bound by their professional code of ethics. As managers, they owe loyalty to the institution that employs them. This can result in a number of ethical dilemmas. A very basic question for the manager is: Which is more important, the patient's well-being or the organization's profit? Can these seemingly opposite responsibilities be reconciled so that both may benefit?

THE MANAGER AS MORAL AGENT

According to Darr,[1] health services managers are moral agents obligated to bring about an ethical environment in which the patient is of prime importance and profit is a secondary concern. Darr feels that managers cannot simply be morally neutral technocrats; the manager must be the organization's conscience. In radiologic technology, Dowd[2] has also stated that patients must be the primary concern, with technical aspects of care a secondary concern. The medical imaging professional could be described as part humanist and part scientist.

Some years ago, it may have been appropriate for the health service manager to view himself or herself as a "hotel" manager, ensuring the survival of the institution, with the ethics of patient care falling to doctors or nurses. This is no longer true. Seiden[3] states that the survival of an institution is important only as long as it serves its societal function. And Summers[4] asks: Is doing good the same as doing well?

The Leadership Factor

Medical imaging needs effective leaders and role models. There is currently a lack of strong leadership in medical imaging and other health professions. Wesbury[5] has argued that the leadership role of managers forces them to consider ethical implications. Levinson[6] states that managers will not succeed if they do not build a consensus of values between the institution and employees.

Summers identifies three questions that a leader must ask to get beyond being merely role-directed (i.e., a morally neutral technocrat): (1) What are my reasons for working in the institution? (2) What does my profession seem to expect of me? and (3) What is the mission of my institution?[4]

> **DISCUSSION QUESTION**
> One of the most difficult issues in the hospital is maintaining a consensus of values between all the different health-care professionals who work there, such as nurses and imaging professionals. How can managers foster an atmosphere of cooperation to ensure quality patient care?

Ethical Pressures and Tasks of a Manager

As leaders, managers face more ethical pressures than staff imagers or other frontline workers might face. To further complicate a manager's task, some of these ethical pressures are in conflict. The conflicting ethical pressures and tasks that a manager must somehow reconcile are as follows:

Pressure	*Task*
Patients	Maximizing health care
Stockholders or owners	Minimizing costs and maximizing profits
Employees	Fair treatment and fair compensation
Upper management	Following directives
Their own careers (internal pressures or egoism)	Egocentric concerns

Patients place ethical pressure on a manager to maximize health care. Stockholders and owners, and their agents (upper management), expect costs to be kept to a minimum in conjunction with expecting maximum profit (or, in the case of a nonprofit health-care institution, minimum charges to patients).[7] Employees expect fair treatment and fair compensation from a manager.[8] Upper managers expect middle managers and frontline managers to follow directives and orders. Finally, managers have pressure arising from concerns for their own well-being and career advancement.

The ethical relationship between a manager and a patient is, in many ways, similar to that of any frontline health-care worker and a patient (see Box 11–1). The relationship is different, however, in that a manager has a very real concern to hold costs to a minimum. These include costs to the patient and to the shareholders (or stakeholders) in an institution.

Employees expect fair treatment and fair compensation from managers. Fair treatment is certainly an ethical pressure. The fair treatment of employees can conflict with the treatment of patients. This is especially true if the institution maintains a strong policy of "The customer (or patient) is always right." A problem can arise here when a patient's demand is unreasonable—

Box 11–1. AMERICAN HOSPITAL ASSOCIATION PATIENT BILL OF RIGHTS

INTRODUCTION

Effective health care requires collaboration between patients and physicians and other health care professionals. Open and honest communication, respect for personal and professional values, and sensitivity to differences are integral to optimal patient care. As the setting for the provision of health services, hospitals must provide a foundation for understanding and respecting the rights and responsibilities of patients, their families, physicians, and other caregivers. Hospitals must ensure a health care ethic that respects the role of patients in decision-making about treatment choices and other aspects of their care. Hospitals must be sensitive to cultural, racial, linguistic, religious, age, gender, and other differences as well as to the needs of persons with disabilities.

The American Hospital Association presents *A Patient's Bill of Rights* with the expectation that it will contribute to more effective patient care and be supported by the hospital on behalf of the institution, its medical staff, employees, and patients. The American Hospital Association encourages health care institutions to tailor this bill of rights to their patient community by translating and/or simplifying the language of this bill of rights as may be necessary to ensure that patients and their families understand their rights and responsibilities.

BILL OF RIGHTS

1. The patient has the right to considerate and respectful care.
2. The patient has the right to and is encouraged to obtain from physicians and other direct caregivers relevant, current, and understandable information concerning diagnosis, treatment, and prognosis.

   Except in emergencies when the patient lacks decision-making capacity and the need for treatment is urgent, the patient is entitled to the opportunity to discuss and request information related to the specific procedures and/or treatments, the risks involved, the possible length of recuperation, and the medically reasonable alternatives and their accompanying risks and benefits.

   Patients have the right to know the identity of physicians, nurses, and others involved in their care, as well as when those involved are students, residents, or other trainees. The patient also has the right to know the immediate and long-term financial implications of treatment choices, insofar as they are known.
3. The patient has the right to make decisions about the plan of care prior to and during the course of treatment and to refuse a recommended treatment or plan of care to the extent permitted by law and hospital policy and to be informed of the medical consequences of this action. In case of such refusal, the patient is entitled to other appropriate care and services that the hospital provides or transfer to another hospital. The hospital should notify patients of any policy that might affect patient choice within the institution.
4. The patient has the right to have an advance directive (such as a living will, health care proxy, or durable power of attorney for health care) concerning treatment or designating a surrogate decision maker with the expectation that the hospital will honor the intent of that directive to the extent permitted by law and hospital policy.

   Health care institutions must advise patients of their rights under state law and hospital policy to make informed medical choices, ask if the patient has an advance directly, and include that information in patient records. The patient has the right to timely information about hospital policy that may limit its ability to implement fully a legally valid advance directive.

5. The patient has the right to every consideration of privacy. Case discussion, consultation, examination, and treatment should be conducted so as to protect each patient's privacy.

6. The patient has the right to expect that all communications and records pertaining to his/her care will be treated as confidential by the hospital, except in cases such as suspected abuse and public health hazards when reporting is permitted or required by law. The patient has the right to expect that the hospital will emphasize the confidentiality of this information when it releases it to any other parties entitled to review information in these records.

7. The patient has the right to review the records pertaining to his/her medical care and to have the information explained or interpreted as necessary, except when restricted by law.

8. The patient has the right to expect that, within its capacity and policies, a hospital will make reasonable response to the request of a patient for appropriate and medically indicated care and services. The hospital must provide evaluation, service, and/or referral as indicated by the urgency of the case. When medically appropriate and legally permissible, or when a patient has so requested, a patient may be transferred to another facility. The institution to which the patient is to be transferred must first have accepted the patient for transfer. The patient must also have the benefit of complete information and explanation concerning the need for, risks, benefits, and alternatives to such a transfer.

9. The patient has the right to ask and be informed of the existence of business relationships among the hospital, educational institutions, other health care providers, or payers that may influence the patient's treatment and care.

10. The patient has the right to consent to or decline to participate in proposed research studies or human experimentation affecting care and treatment or requiring direct patient involvement, and to have those studies fully explained prior to consent. A patient who declines to participate in research or experimentation is entitled to the most effective care that the hospital can otherwise provide.

11. The patient has the right to expect reasonable continuity of care when appropriate and to be informed by physicians and other caregivers of available and realistic patient care options when hospital care is no longer appropriate.

12. The patient has the right to be informed of hospital policies and practices that relate to patient care, treatment, and responsibilities. The patient has the right to be informed of available resources for resolving disputes, grievances, and conflicts, such as ethics committees, patient representatives, or other mechanisms available in the institution. The patient has the right to be informed of the hospital's charges for services and available payment methods. The collaborative nature of health care requires that patients, or their families/surrogates, participate in their care. The effectiveness of care and patient satisfaction with the course of treatment depend, in part, on the patient fulfilling certain responsibilities. Patients are responsible for providing information about past illnesses, hospitalizations, medications, and other matters related to health status. To participate effectively in decision-making, patients must be encouraged to take responsibility for requesting additional information or clarification about their health status or treatment when they do not fully understand information and instructions. Patients are also responsible

for ensuring that the health care institution has a copy of their written advance directive if they have one. Patients are responsible for informing their physicians and other caregivers if they anticipate problems in following prescribed treatment.

Patients should also be aware of the hospital's obligation to be reasonably efficient and equitable in providing care to other patients and the community. The hospital's rules and regulations are designed to help the hospital meet this obligation. Patients and their families are responsible for making reasonable accommodations to the needs of the hospital, other patients, medical staff, and hospital employees. Patients are responsible for providing necessary information for insurance claims and for working with the hospital to make payment arrangements, when necessary.

A person's health depends on much more than health care services. Patients are responsible for recognizing the impact of their lifestyle on their personal health.

CONCLUSION

Hospitals have many functions to perform, including the enhancement of health status, health promotions, and the prevention and treatment of injury and disease; the immediate and ongoing care and rehabilitation of patients; the education of health professionals, patients, and the community; and research. All these activities must be conducted with an overriding concern for the values and dignity of patients.

Reprinted with permission from the American Hospital Association

which, while rare, does happen. The manager must then decide what is fair and ethical.

A more obvious ethical dilemma for a manager arises from employee expectations of fair compensation and the conflicting expectations of patients and stockholders or owners. Higher compensation for employees will make them happy, but it will leave less money for equipment that serves the patients or profits for shareholders. On the other hand, a problem may result when too little compensation is offered. Although this may satisfy the need to minimize costs, it may compromise patient care because only low-skill workers will accept low wages.

> **DISCUSSION QUESTION**
> What are the wages for radiographers and other imaging professionals in your area? Do you consider these fair wages? What factors influence wages? List five factors a manager must consider when determining the appropriate wage for a professional worker.

Upper management exerts pressure on managers to obey orders and directives. Directives to reduce staff can violate an ethical duty to employees and patients. Poor directives may result in waste and compromise an ethical duty to owners and shareholders. Orders to ignore or cover up mismanagement and mistakes can violate a manager's personal ethics. It is difficult for a manager to choose between what he or she believes to be right and what his or her boss has commanded.

Finally, managers have egocentric concerns. We are familiar with the manager or businessperson, as portrayed in the movies, who is concerned only with short-term gain and personal profit. If managers do not address and resolve their egoistic ethics, then their endeavors may be either amoral or immoral.[9]

DISCUSSION QUESTION
A group of medical imaging managers sold outdated and exposed x-ray film to reclaim the silver (a common practice) but, opting for short-term gain, underreported the amount in collusion with their company. These managers received a kickback for doing so. What ethical principles did these managers violate? What is the best means of preventing incidents like this from occurring?

APPLICATION OF ETHICAL PRINCIPLES TO MANAGEMENT

This section discusses the basic ethical principles of beneficence and nonmaleficence; autonomy, confidentiality, and informed consent (respect for people); veracity; and justice as they relate to the role of a manager. These theoretical principles, discussed earlier in the book, have practical implications in the management of health-care facilities, including imaging services.

Beneficence and Nonmaleficence

Beneficence refers to doing good. The primary beneficiary of a manager's good should be the patient, although, as noted earlier, there are often multiple beneficiaries to be considered: the physician, the institution (and perhaps its stockholders), and the community. The concepts of beneficence and nonmaleficence have their roots in the Hippocratic Oath.

The practice of beneficence can be related to the risk-benefit consideration made in radiation exposure. Patients should undergo radiologic examinations only when the potential benefit outweighs the potential risk of the procedure. The potential benefit is beneficence (doing good); the potential risk is maleficence (doing harm).

If a health-care professional can do no good for the patient, at the very least no harm should be done. A strong administrative obligation to bring

TABLE 11–1
DIFFERENCES BETWEEN LAW AND ETHICS

Law	Ethics
Focuses on "shall nots"	Focuses on "shalls" or "shoulds"
Implemented at a societal level	Most often a personal choice
Minimum standard for societal morality	Higher calling; more demanding than law
Should reflect overall ethics of society; may, however, represent special interests	Forces consideration of disparate views and needs

about nonmaleficence is to ensure that staff are competent and that appropriate safety measures are taken. Laws to ensure safety are only the first step; managers who practice nonmaleficence only to the extent that laws and regulations require are using law as a refuge for their own lack of ethics.[6] Differences between law and ethics are summarized in Table 11–1.

Autonomy, Confidentiality, and Informed Consent

Three interrelated concepts involve respect for people: autonomy, or the capacity for self-direction; the preservation of patient confidentiality and privacy, difficult in an information society; and informed consent. In an increasingly privatized and competitive market, in which, Michelman[10] states, "respect for others has no place," managers must take extra care to observe respect for people.

Autonomy

A manager has the obligation to bring about continued growth of staff, fostering increased autonomy through staff development. Staff development is growth-oriented, provides opportunity for self-direction, integrates the needs of the learner (employee) and facility, focuses on the long term, and shares decision making between management and employees. Only recently has this need been recognized; in imaging departments, it was assumed that the staff possessed skills that were adequate for the short term and easily modifiable for the long term.[11] Drafke[12] had to invent a new term—managee— for his text on health-care administration and the role of the employee because previous terms all tended to negate the employee's autonomy.

Humans are paradoxical creatures who seek independence while retaining dependency needs.[13] Sometimes employees clamor for more responsibility and then, when it is offered, withdraw into a shell of complacency. Although this is frustrating for the manager, it does not minimize the obligation to bring about growth.

**Box 11–2. AMERICAN HEALTH INFORMATION
MANAGERS ASSOCIATION GUIDELINES FOR THE USE
OF THE FAX MACHINE**

1. Patient data should be faxed only when the original document or mail-delivered copies will not serve the intended purpose.
2. Patient data should be faxed only when the information will be used for patient care. It should *not* be used for routine release of data to insurance companies, attorneys, or other entities who may be served as well with other carriers.
3. Authorization should be secured before releasing any information; this includes the development of proper guidelines for the release of data in emergency situations.
4. Users must be trained in proper procedure.
5. Fax machines should be located in secure locations.
6. Fax records must comply with guidelines such as accreditation standards, federal and state laws for maintaining medical records, and state statutes for the admissibility of records as evidence.
7. Misdirected faxes should be directed to the risk manager, and the site receiving a misdirected fax should be instructed to destroy it.

Confidentiality and Privacy

Although the need for confidentiality is easy to understand, it is difficult to maintain in the medical environment, especially with advances in technology. Rowan[14] states that it becomes easy for health-care professionals to forget the importance of privacy because they so often see patients at a time when the patients are powerless and vulnerable. However, patients who feel that their right to privacy has been violated will not return to the institution that has violated it, or may feel compelled to sue for breach of care.[15]

Confidentiality can be breached through careless speech and careless use of technology. Grumbine[16] feels that "elevator talk" is the most common spoken breach of confidentiality. Other breaches may result from the use of paging phones in the cafeteria, the discussion of medical images in a reading area (where patients can often overhear), and the verbal reading of reports over the phone by transcriptionists (although allowed, this may lead to a breach of confidentiality if the individual receiving the information poses as an authorized receiver).

The photocopier, which makes it almost *too* easy to make copies, is a big culprit in the breach of confidentiality; records are sometimes left in the copier. The fax machine, although a boon for the rapid transmission of information, is fast becoming the biggest culprit in violating patient privacy; faxes may be misdirected. The American Health Information Managers Association (AHIMA) has developed guidelines for the use of the fax machine (Box 11–2).[17]

The final breach of confidentiality may occur with increased dependence on computer networks and databases and the subsequent potential for misuse of computer records. Employees may also be tempted to access information that they should not access, such as the status of a neighbor.

To help maintain confidentiality, there should be regular education of the staff. Facilities should also have confidentiality committees to evaluate procedures for maintaining confidentiality, especially as it is affected by new technology.

Informed Consent

Managers are responsible for ensuring that policies for obtaining informed consent are established within their departments. Although physicians are responsible for obtaining informed consent, managers need to ensure that such policies are in place and are being implemented and that all employees understand how they work.

Another issue is the representation of medical imaging on institutional review boards (IRBs). In the past, the involvement of medical imaging professionals in research has been limited, and primarily physicians, PhD researchers, and nurses were represented on IRBs. As this changes, these professionals should ensure that they participate in IRB approval; a logical choice is the department manager.

Veracity

Veracity is truthfulness. Health-care professionals are not allowed to lie to the patient. Even so-called benevolent lying to spare the patient from pain is not acceptable. Patients, once they realize that some health-care professionals are lying to them, will no longer trust health-care professionals as a group. For medical treatment to be successful, trust in the health-care worker is absolutely necessary.

Managers must also be truthful with their employees. Again, once an employee no longer trusts a manager, he or she will no longer work in the same fashion. The manager who cannot be trusted cannot expect loyalty from employees.

Justice

Justice holds that fairness and impartiality should prevail. Decisions should reflect equality for all. This includes the allocation of medical resources, which Seiden[3] believes to be one of the primary ethical dilemmas faced by health-care managers. Bader and Burness[18] note, "Dollars spent on one expensive technology cannot be spent on something else." For example, the medical imaging manager might be confronted with an ethical dilemma in the decision to buy a new MRI scanner when it is obvious that it is not needed. The money could be better spent elsewhere; however, a push is on to be the only hospital in town with this new scanner to maintain a competitive edge.

Although current debates on the rationing of health care in the United States often seem to assume that health care is *not* already rationed, in fact it is. The dominant method of rationing health care in the United States is the merit (also known as "price" or "laissez-faire") method. In this method, limited resources are rationed on the basis of who can afford them, with some resources available on a charity basis.[19] The privatization and competitive basis for health care begun in the 1980s has taken firm root.

In the 1940s, Sister J. Gabriel[20] could state that "a hospital's obligation to its community is not measured by its net earnings, but by the services it renders, regardless of whether the community pays for such service or not." Now a manager must often consider obligations to a group of shareholders as well as to the patient. Some years ago Relman[21] wrote that the developing "medical-industrial complex" is

> . . . more efficient than its non-profit competition, but it creates the problems of overuse and fragmentation of services, overemphasis on technology, and "cream skimming," and it may also exercise undue influence on national health policy. Closer attention from the public and the profession, and careful study, are necessary to ensure that the "medical-industrial complex" puts the interests of the public before those of its stockholders.

DISCUSSION QUESTION

Which type of rationing of health care do you support? Why? What are the positive aspects of the U.S. system? What are its negative aspects? How could U.S. health care be improved? Should managers support any one type of rationing? Why or why not?

Many institutions can deliver outstanding patient care. The difficulty lies in providing good care for a reasonable cost. The pressure to provide the utmost in patient diagnosis and treatment is in conflict with the pressures to hold down costs and increase profits (or reduce charges). Recent concerns for governmental reform of health care is due to a perception that health-care costs have *not* been controlled in the past.

The stockholders or owners of any health-care institution expect managers to do everything possible to care for patients *and* keep costs at a minimum. Waste is to be eliminated, of course. However, stockholders and owners expect that legitimate spending and employee salaries be kept as low as possible. These expectations can conflict with those of patients and of employees. Patient care may be compromised sometimes for the sake of saving a buck, but more commonly, patients are inconvenienced. For example, hiring more staff members and purchasing more equipment may ensure that patients are cared for immediately. However, a manager would be violating the ethic expected from owners and stockholders. Conversely, a manager may have minimal staff and be saving money, only to have extremely long patient waiting times. Managers must then compromise both. The difficulty is that there is no one right answer as to how many people to hire or how long patients should wait.

> **DISCUSSION QUESTION**
> One aspect of holding down costs involves working with physicians who insist that certain pieces of equipment are essential to delivering quality care. Often new techniques appear in journals that require new equipment (e.g., new catheters in the cardiac catheterization laboratory). How does a manager balance the demands of physicians with the needs of stockholders and patients to hold costs to a minimum? At what point should the manager say no?

CONCLUSION

Managers have a number of responsibilities. For the manager to function effectively as a professional, the various ethical pressures and tasks of a manager must be considered, as well as the need to follow ethical principles. As moral agents and leaders for the imaging professions, managers must reconcile responsibility with their own need to succeed (egoism). As professionals, managers must ensure that patients are the primary beneficiaries of health care, while remembering that profit drives the current health-care system. This gives the imaging manager a number of challenging ethical problems and dilemmas to deal with on a daily basis.

REFERENCES

1. Darr, K: Patient-centered ethics for health services managers. Journal of Health and Human Resources Administration 16(2):197–216, 1993.
2. Dowd, SB: The radiographers' role: Part scientist, part humanist. Radiol Technol 63(4):240–243, 1992.
3. Seiden, DJ: Ethics for hospital administrators. Hospital and Health Services Administration 1983, 28(2):81–89, 1983.
4. Summers, JW: Doing good and doing well: Ethics, professionalism, and success. Hospital and Health Services Administration 29(2):84–100, 1984.
5. Wesbury, SA: Ethics in health services administration: A case for constant reevaluation. The Eight Annual Reverend J. Flanagan SJ Lecture in Hospital Administration. St. Louis, March 19, 1980.
6. Levinson, H: The changing role of the hospital administrator. Health Care Manage Rev 1(1):79, 1979.
7. Ferrell, OC, and Gardner, G: In Pursuit of Ethics: Tough Choices in the World of Business. Springfield, Ill, Smith Collins, 1991.

8. Pride, WN, Hughes, R, and Kapoor, J: Business ed 4. Boston, Houghton Mifflin, 1993.
9. Bucholz, R: Fundamental Concepts and Problems in Business Ethics. Englewood Cliffs, NJ, Prentice-Hall, 1989.
10. Michelman, JH: Some ethical consequences of economic competition. Journal of Business Ethics 2:79–87, 1983.
11. Dowd, SB: Integrating the needs of the individual and institution in staff development. Radiology Management 15(1):33, 1992.
12. Drafke, MW: Working in Health Care: What You Need to Know to Succeed. Philadelphia, FA Davis, 1994.
13. Smith, RM: Learning How To Learn: Applied Theory for Adults. Englewood Cliffs, NJ, Cambridge Adult Education, 1982.
14. Rowan, K: Hospital patients have a right to privacy. RN 56:92, 1993.
15. Dowd, SB, and Dowd, LP: Confidentiality issues for healthcare professionals. Today's Ethics Journal, in press.
16. Grumbine, DA: Revisiting confidentiality. Radiology Management 16:35, 1994.
17. Koska, MT: Outcomes research: Hospitals face confidentiality concerns. Hospitals 66:32, 1992 (January, 5).
18. Bader, BS, and Burness, A. Ethics: Boards address issues beyond allocation of resources. Trustee 35:14, 1982.
19. Hiller, MD: Ethics and health care administration: Issues in education and practice. The Journal of Health Administration Education 2(2):147–192, 1984.
20. Gabriel, J: The hospital and the changing social order. In Bachmeyer, AC, and Hartman, G (eds), The Hospital in Modern Society. New York, Commonwealth Fund, 1943. p 19.
21. Relman, AS. The new medical-industrial complex. N Engl J Med 303:963, 1983.

Index

An "f" following a page number indicates a figure. A "t" indicates a table.